ADVERSE CHILDHOOD EXPERIENCES

This guide provides healthcare students and professionals with a foundational background on adverse childhood experiences (ACEs) – traumatic early life experiences, which can have a profound impact on health in later life.

ACEs can include being a victim of abuse, neglect or exposure to risk in the home or community. How healthcare students and professionals learn to recognize, react and respond to persons affected by trauma will lay the foundation for their relationships with patients. This book intentionally uses micro-to-macro lenses accompanied by a structural competency framework to elucidate health implications across the lifespan. It explores the nature of adversity and its effects on the physical, emotional, cognitive and social health of individuals, communities and society. The book, written by two experienced psychiatric nurses, will equip healthcare students and professionals with an understanding for critical change in practice and offer action steps designed to assist them with prevention and intervention approaches and steps to help build resilience.

This book will be core reading for healthcare students within mental health, pediatric and primary care nursing courses. It will also be of interest to students and professionals in the social work, psychology and public health fields who are exploring resilience and trauma-informed practices.

Roberta Waite is a Professor at Drexel University, College of Nursing and Health Professions and Assistant Dean of Academic and Community Integration at the Stephen and Sandra Sheller Eleventh Street Family Health Services of Drexel University.

Ruth Ann Ryan is a Board Certified Clinical Nurse Specialist and a Psychoeducation Training Specialist with the Healing Hurt People Program in the Center for Non-Violence and Social Justice at Drexel University College of Medicine. She is co-founder of the Sanctuary Model and was the Clinical Director of the program for 20 years.

ADVERSE CHILDHOOD EXPERIENCES

What Students and Health Professionals Need to Know

Roberta Waite and Ruth Ann Ryan

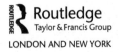
Routledge
Taylor & Francis Group

LONDON AND NEW YORK

First published 2020
by Routledge
2 Park Square, Milton Park, Abingdon, Oxon OX14 4RN

and by Routledge
52 Vanderbilt Avenue, New York, NY 10017

Routledge is an imprint of the Taylor & Francis Group, an informa business

British Library Cataloguing in Publication Data
A catalogue record for this book is available from the British Library

Library of Congress Cataloging-in-Publication Data
A catalog record has been requested for this book

ISBN: 978-0-367-20378-8 (hbk)
ISBN: 978-0-367-20382-5 (pbk)
ISBN: 978-0-429-26120-6 (ebk)

Typeset in Bembo
by Taylor & Francis Books

CONTENTS

ILLUSTRATIONS

Figures

Tables

Boxes

ABOUT THE AUTHORS

Roberta Waite, EdD, PMHCNS, ANEF, FAAN is a Professor at Drexel University, College of Nursing and Health Professions and Assistant Dean of Academic and Community Integration at the Stephen and Sandra Sheller Eleventh Street Family Health Services of Drexel University. As an advanced practice psychiatric nurse, her scholarship and research centers on behavioral health concerns, specifically adult ADHD, psychological trauma, and depression and their effects on health outcomes as well as promoting systemic prevention/ early intervention efforts. Dr. Waite's educational research focuses on leadership development of students in the health professions and public health while concurrently fostering critical consciousness using a social justice lens.

Ruth Ann Ryan, MSN, CS is a Board Certified Clinical Nurse Specialist and a Psychoeducation Training Specialist with the Healing Hurt People Program in the Center for Non-Violence and Social Justice at Drexel University College of Medicine. She is co- founder of the Sanctuary Model and was the Clinical Director of the program for 20 years. She and her colleagues developed the S.E.L.F. Model of trauma recovery, which has been implemented in programs for children, adolescents and adults in many national and international locations. Ruth Ann has 30 years of experience in the trauma field as a psychotherapist and organizational consultant on trauma informed principles and practices. She co-authored a group manual titled, *S.E.L.F.: A Trauma-Informed Psychoeducational Group Curriculum* and has been training on this model in educational settings and clinical programs throughout the United States.

PART I

Knowledge development about ACEs

1

INTRODUCTION

Repression to spoken truth – Opening up

The theme of this chapter is reflective of a saying by Bessel A. van der Kolk, "As long as you keep secrets and suppress information, you are fundamentally at war with yourself . . . The critical issue is allowing yourself to know what you know. That takes an enormous amount of courage" (Goodreads, 2018, ¶ 2). Both authors share their initial journey to understanding ACEs.

The link to ACEs: Roberta Waite

The question of how to understand the experiences, perspectives, and health beliefs about depression from the lens of self-identified African American women led me on a journey of conducting research exploring the cultural nature of depression. In doing so, it was in 2005 that I encountered the unfurling manifestation of the human narrative. The voices of courageous women who took part in this research showed me there exist parts of individuals' life stories that will disturb and alarm even the most intrepid researcher. The social meaning and contextually-based accounts of depression, the framework used to make sense of these experiences, past events, and the complexities of connecting with others in addition to the consequences of such interaction were shared. As an advanced practice nurse researcher, women's subjective experience about depression revealed an unexpected theme—never voiced childhood adversity. In living with depression, women revealed what was salient in their life experience through telling their story. Open, authentic sharing among the women fostered a culture of safety allowing deep-seated experiences to surface. No direct question about abuse was posed; however one focus group participant uttered her experience of abuse, specifically sexual abuse by a family member. Several other participants were able to share deeply-rooted unspoken truths of their own. Beliefs about the cause(s) of depression were likely a stimulating factor. Interestingly, each woman believed they were the only ones who had experienced such tragedy during their earlier years of life. These thoughts were so taboo they had repressed them for years. Many perceived that what was not spoken was known among family members but never voiced. This entrenched the notion of *knowing and not knowing about the elephant in the room*. Few had shared these experiences with anyone, including their primary care provider. Their constructed narrative presented events that were part of their world and discernments about these events.

Adverse early life experiences, as a fundamental theme of this qualitative research, drove my desire to want to learn more about how this phenomenon impacted the lives of these women, especially as it related to their health. My journey through graduate school to earn a Master's Degree as an advanced practice adult psychiatric nurse in 1993 did not expose me to the link between early life experiences and health in later life. Hoping to understand more about this connection, I dug deeper and in the process learned of a training taking place at the Behavioral Health Training and Education Network (BHTEN) in Philadelphia, Pennsylvania entitled "Trauma Theory 101: What Everyone Needs to Know About the Impact of Trauma, Adversity and Toxic Stress," led by Dr. Sandra Bloom, an activist and Board Certified Psychiatrist. Well, everything changed from this point forward. This was a great touchstone moment for me. Gaining awareness about a framework to situate information learned from women who were able to dive deep into their unconscious and reveal deeply-repressed feelings aligns with the revolutionary research undertaken by Dr. Felitti and Dr. Anda—The Adverse Childhood Experiences Study. As part of their journey, many women who engaged in the research study came to realize pearls of self-discovery and personal liberation. The repressed feelings were given air to breathe and they no longer had to deny their personal wounds.

The link to ACEs: Ruth Ann Ryan

My journey to the co-authorship of this book began over three decades ago when, equipped with a newly earned Master's Degree in Nursing with a focus in family systems, I was fortunate to be invited to join a small, multidisciplinary team charged with the task of starting a mental health in-patient unit in a small rural general hospital. It was an opportunity to engage in a creative endeavor with team members who became lifelong colleagues and friends. When Sandy Bloom, MD and Joe Foderaro, LCSW and I began our work we had no notion that along the way, our clients would awaken us to their life stories of trauma and resilience and teach us about the profoundly important need to understand health and well-being through a very different lens than we had been schooled in. My work at what became the Sanctuary Programs, which existed for 20 years throughout the 1980s and 1990s, changed me both professionally and personally and shifted my medical model perspective on health to a trauma-informed perspective. My lens changed, becoming a much more wide-angle one that incorporated a deeper understanding of the many ways in which context is at play as a determinant of health.

The awakening was painful; the stories of our clients were filled with brutal examples of human suffering emanating from the misuse and abuse of power and control. Our work preceded the adverse childhood experiences (ACEs) study but our clinical practice produced what we called practice-based evidence of the consequences of adversity, chronic stress and abuse. It became clear that, if healing was to take place and if health was to be restored, health care delivery had to radically change and, as my colleague simply and eloquently stated years ago, the question had to shift from "what is wrong with people to what has happened to them?" I felt compelled to learn more, to speak out about all that I was learning and do what I could to share the developing knowledge about human induced trauma and its consequences. Along the way, the lens kept widening as the realizations about context grew to include treatment settings and the often-inadvertent ways they replicate power abuses. The lens eventually encompassed and implicated financial and societal structures that do the same. It became clear to me that this wealth of information must be understood and integrated into the education and practice of health care professionals so that our shared work could bring about change.

We share these stories to demonstrate how the spoken truth about trauma can start a movement where individuals no longer have to be silent. *Speaking truth to power* is extremely germane for individuals who share their story openly, given the courage it takes to open up and no longer repress the truth about their experience. It is up to all of us, especially health professionals, to more fully understand the phenomenon of trauma and push back on those structures, systems of oppression, and people that sanction silence about these issues by not making this information integral to didactic and clinical education, research, and practice. As experts of their own life experience, individuals we encounter who have experienced trauma deserve nothing less than our best to support their healing.

Reflecting on these significant issues brings realization to the critical need to empower students and individuals working in the health professions to become knowledgeable about ACEs. We cannot address this issue effectively and promote hope and healing if we first do not engage in knowledge development about ACEs including understanding their impact from a life course health development perspective. How health professions students and graduates of these disciplines recognize, react, and respond to persons affected by trauma lays the foundation for relationships formed. During our professional experience, we have frequently seen the shame, isolation, and individualistic approach to healing due to professionals' lack of knowledge and adeptness of skill in the related area. Moreover, lack of understanding about trauma and its association with oppression will also be explored. Countering the narrative of blame as well as identity of someone living in existence of wounded-ness and poor health requires the attention of all health professionals. Therefore, ACEs curriculum must be infused throughout students' academic learning. Seeing the excitement of brain science, especially how the plasticity of the brain can affect health outcomes related to trauma and healing, offers hope regarding prevention efforts that should take a social-ecological approach. We will examine this content and the associated effects when this is not recognized, which contributes to a lifetime of emotional, behavioral, and medical symptoms and diagnoses. Readers will learn about models of care that help to mitigate trauma and promote resiliency and models of care that risk possible cover for the status quo. The individual emphasis on promoting wellness and resiliency is far too common, requiring individuals to respond and cope generally from within. As readers learn about translating trauma-informed care into improving practice, its effects on families will be reviewed. By using the universal paradigm of implementing trauma-informed practice when engaging others, health professionals will be applying an intervention useful to everyone. ACEs are widespread, long-lasting, and do not discriminate, which is evident given the extensive prevalence of present-day trauma in the lives of individuals, families, and communities worldwide. Taking steps to not be complicit in driving the ignorance regarding ACEs is no longer acceptable, nor is it an option. Knowledge development readers will gain, and action steps they should take, will be outlined in this book to better equip individuals to determine the charge they will take to address ACEs from intrapersonal, interpersonal, communal, and societal levels.

2

MAKING THE CONNECTION

The ACE study

Background: Original ACE study

The history of the Adverse Childhood Experiences (ACE) Study serves as a forewarning for many individuals in the health professions. Dr. Felitti, an internist, practicing at the Department of Preventative Medicine at Kaiser Permanente in San Diego, California uncovered that significant adversity in childhood was precluding many of his morbidly obese clients from maintaining their weight loss (Felitti, 2002). By understanding the distant root causes of maladaptation and by exposing the adversities that may perhaps lead to behavioral allostasis (i.e. behaviors that blunt the stress response), professionals are better situated to establish strong therapeutic relationships, to empower clients with a more profound understanding regarding why they might feel trapped in unhealthy behaviors. Also, professionals with insight into root causes of maladaptation are better able to support a person's progression toward healing and managing more adaptively moving forward (Garner, 2016). These conceptualizations are integral as we peer into what ACEs are as well as ACE-related behaviors that can have life-long consequences. The co-authors assert that awareness and recognition of ACEs is paramount in order to change the paradigm of practice for those in the health professions.

In 1985, Dr. Felitti was working with individuals suffering from obesity and who were striving to lose weight through his Positive Choice Program (Stiles, 2003). He made an unusual clinical observation in that individuals in the weight loss program who accomplished the most success were similarly most liable to drop out of the weight loss program. This conundrum led him to dig deeper regarding participants' behavior. Additional questioning and detailed interviews of over 200 program participants led Dr. Felitti to uncover a central theme among the group—child abuse was extraordinarily commonplace in the lives of his participants and the abuse characteristically preceded development of obesity (Felitti, 2002). Dr. Felitti uncovered the link by mistake while questioning one of the members who dropped out of the weight loss program. It was during the interview that the woman self-confessed to initially being sexually active when she weighed around 40 pounds. She further elucidated that she was merely four years of age and the sexual activity was initiated by her father (Murphy, Fiorillo, & Sullivan, 2014).

Consequently, realization that obesity was not the real problem was counterintuitive. Actually, participants in the weight loss program used obesity as the remedy for managing more catastrophic struggles—not being able to give voice to and gain treatment for deep-seated injuries (trauma). The social taboo, shame and secrecy of traumatic life experiences during childhood and adolescence were hidden by time but continued to wreak havoc on the lives of those affected. Obesity served as a protectant for them, a form of self-preservation; individuals in this weight loss program felt securer being larger versus normal size because they would be less desirable or more feared due to size. There was also fearfulness of change (Felitti, 2002).

Pursuant to these novel findings, Felitti spoke at the North American Association for the Study of Obesity sharing the frequent association between obesity and abusive childhood experiences. This meeting occurred in Atlanta and consequently employees from the Centers for Disease Control and Prevention (CDC) attended which led to the connection of Dr. Felitti with Dr. Robert Anda and Dr. David Williamson, senior researchers in Preventive Medicine and Epidemiology at the CDC. CDC researchers realized the significance of what had been reported which led to the sponsorship of a large epidemiologic study now known as the ACE Study. These three doctors (Felitti, Williamson and Anda) and their colleagues started a blueprint for the criteria to be used for the ACE Study in order to understand how childhood events can affect adult health (Murphy et al., 2014). This was a formidable partnership since Kaiser's Department of Preventive Medicine provided an ideal setting carrying out at one site comprehensive biomedical, psychological, and social (biopsychosocial) evaluations. The CDC would play an integral part with the study design and massive data management needed for meaningful interpretation of clinical observations. The study was intended to respond to the question: "If risk factors for disease, disability, and early mortality are not randomly distributed, what early life influences precede the adoption or development of them?" (Murphy et al., 2014, p. 5).

Through Kaiser Permanente, the largest prepaid, non-profit, health care delivery system in the United States, over 26,000 consecutive adults who received services in the Department of Preventive Medicine were asked if they would be interested in taking part in a study to help gain a better understanding of how childhood events may affect adult health status. Interestingly, 68% of adults receiving services consented to participate and after specific exclusions for incomplete data and duplicate contributions, the ACE Study included an estimated 17,000 individuals (Leitch, 2017). All participants were informed that the data they offered about their childhood would be separate from their medical records. Researchers at the CDC designed the research protocols that would compare current adult health status to childhood experiences decades earlier with individuals who received services at the Department of Preventive Medicine. This study, consisting of surveys and exams, was conducted at Kaiser Permanente in two waves running from 1995 to 1997 and participants were followed for about 15 years (Murphy et al., 2014). With the surveys, each research participant supplied detailed data about their childhood experiences of abuse, family dysfunction, neglect, as well as their current health status and behaviors. Eight categories of adverse childhood experiences were included in the initial survey including three forms of abuse (sexual, verbal, and physical) and five forms of family dysfunction (a parent who was an alcoholic or mentally ill, a mother who was the victim of domestic violence, a family member who had been incarcerated, and the loss of a parent through divorce or abandonment). Subsequently, emotional neglect and physical neglect were included in the second wave of the survey (Murphy et al., 2014). Consequently, this totaled 10 ACE categories. Therefore, the ACE score (or adversity score) ranged from zero to ten. If an individual was physically abused hundreds of times during his or her childhood, and did not experience any other category of childhood trauma, the ACE score is one point. Furthermore, if an individual experienced emotional abuse, lived with a mentally ill father, and a mother who was battered, the ACE score is three points. Similarly, an ACE score of six consists of any six of the categories The ACEs questionnaire can be accessed at https://acestoohigh.com/got-your-ace-score/

Questions for the ACE study were constructed from literature reviews, selected questions from published surveys, discussion with experienced researchers, previous research that exhibited these experiences to have significant adverse health or social implications, and they were the most frequently cited factors by a group of an estimated 300 Kaiser Permanente members (Murphy et al., 2014; Leitch, 2017). Notably, all questions were retrospective in nature, reporting incidents of adverse childhood experiences that occurred before 18 years of age. In addition to ACE questions, participants were asked about their health history. The names of the two questionnaires were the Family Health History Questionnaire and the Health Appraisal Questionnaire; there is a male and female version (Centers for Disease Control and Prevention, 2016; access to questionnaires is available at https://www.cdc.gov/violenceprevention/acestudy/about.html).

Of the estimated 17,000 Kaiser Permanente member participants, most were middle-class, college educated, white Americans whose mean age was 56 years and average age was 57 years. There was limited racial diversity—80% white including Hispanic, 10% Black, and 10% Asian. Nearly half of the participants were men (46%) and half were women (54%). The majority of participants had some form of post-secondary education—39% graduated from college and 36% had some college education. Just 7% lacked a high school education. All had high quality health insurance. Interestingly, these participants were from a population traditionally not considered at risk for ACEs (Leitch, 2017).

The language used to name the study was intentional. Dr. Anda and Dr. Felitti chose the term *adverse* because it did not conjure up biased notions about the offenders or victims of child abuse, domestic violence, or persons with mental health or substance abuse problems (Anda, n.d.). Similarly, *adverse* denotes stress which is relevant since the biologic stress response is fundamentally accountable for the negative effect of ACEs on brain development. As indicated by the study, *childhood* signifies the first 17 years of life (Anda, n.d.). Finally, the term *experiences* was selected instead of environment since the latter phrase can infer exposure to environmental toxins (Anda, n.d.).

Findings

What Felitti and Anda discovered from the data collected was unexpected yet pivotal to knowledge development about ACEs and its correlation to health later in life. Specifically, they discovered that ACEs are a central determinant of the health and social well-being of the nation. The scoring showed that one-third of the participants in the original ACE Study had an ACE score of 0. Moreover, if any one ACE category was reported, there was an 87% probability that at least one additional ACE category would exist (Murphy et al., 2014). Furthermore, one in six people indicated an ACE score of 4 or more and participants with this ACE score had a 240% greater risk of hepatitis and sexually transmitted disease, were 460% more likely to experience depression, and were 390% more likely to have chronic obstructive pulmonary disease compared to persons with an ACE score of zero (Murphy et al., 2014). In addition, participants with an ACE score of four or more were twice as likely to be smokers, seven times more likely to be an alcoholic, ten times more likely to have injected street drugs, twelve times more likely to have attempted suicide compared to individuals with an ACE score of zero (Murphy et al., 2014). As well, one in ten individuals reported an ACE score of five or more (Murphy et al., 2014). This means that 10% of the 17,000 research participants, specifically 1,700 people, had been exposed to five or more of these categories of ACEs (Fulford, 2017). The referenced ACE categories (abuse, neglect, and household dysfunction) and their associated prevalence for each area in the study are indicated below:

Abuse

- Emotional—recurrent humiliation (11%)
- Physical—beating, not spanking (28%)
- Contact sexual abuse (28% women, 16% men; 22% overall)

Neglect

- Physical (10%)
- Emotional (15%)

Household dysfunction

- Mother treated violently (13%)
- Household member was alcoholic or drug user (27%)
- Household member was imprisoned (6%)
- Household member was chronically depressed, suicidal, mentally ill, in psychiatric hospital (17%)
- Not raised by both biological parents (23%)

(Anda & Felitti, 2008)

Outcomes from this study highlight that even among a middle class, well-off population with health insurance, we cannot overlook ACEs and we cannot solely base it on stereotypical populations (low-income, racial and ethnic minority groups). We can clearly translate this data into action to create change that can optimize health of diverse populations. Of note, women were 50% more likely than men to report five or more ACEs, which raises inquiry about women's proclivity to unclear health problems (e.g., fibromyalgia, chronic non-malignant pain syndromes, and irritable bowel syndrome). These medical concerns may well be artifacts caused by blindness of practitioners to social realities and ignorance of the impact of gender (Fulford, 2017). Incorporating aspects of ACEs into one's diagnostic and treatment plan formulation may not be a comfortable situation for some, given that it shows how our consideration of ailments is characteristically fixated on tertiary consequences (Felitti, 2002). Often primary issues contributing to ailments are shielded to a large extent by social convention and taboo. Health professionals frequently caring for individuals have limited themselves to the minutest portion of the problem; specifically, that portion they are most comfortable addressing (Felitti, 2002). It's also important for health professionals to realize that outcomes show that ACEs occur in clusters; if one ACE is reported then it is necessary to inquire if other ACEs have occurred (Fulford, 2017). Accordingly, it is evident that every health care professional likely sees individuals in practice with several high ACE scores daily. Characteristically, these may be some of the more challenging individuals practitioners encounter in their daily work.

In summary, the landmark Adverse Childhood Experiences Study discovered a strong graded relationship between the magnitude of exposure to abuse, neglect or household dysfunction during childhood and numerous risk factors for some of the principal causes of death in adulthood. Irrefutably, ACEs are astonishingly common, though normally concealed and unrecognized. ACEs unquestionably have a great effect on individuals' lives decades after these horrific incidents have occurred, although these events are now altered from psychosocial occurrences into organic disease(s), social malfunction, and mental afflictions. Outcomes from the ACE Study must be used as insight given our awareness of its strong correlation to risky health behaviors (e.g., alcohol and drug abuse, obesity, smoking, and sexual risk behaviors), chronic health conditions (e.g., ischemic heart disease, coronary obstructive pulmonary disease, and liver disease), low life potential (e.g., depression, suicide, and work absenteeism), as well as early death (CDC, 2016). With increased numbers of ACEs, risk for these outcomes is enhanced (CDC, 2016). The numerous articles published from the original ACE study can be located on the CDC website: http://www.cdc.gov/violenceprevention/acestudy/journal.html While the ACE study has generated numerous publications and created significant intellectual appeal in the United States and Europe over the past decade, its discoveries have not been transformed into meaningful clinical, educational, or social action or policy change (Anda & Felitti, 2008). As you read this book our hope is that momentum can be developed to make effective change, especially from an educational and practice perspective.

Expanded ACEs

"Human life cannot be studied without taking into account both how individuals are situated within and constrained by social structures and how those individuals construct an understanding of and impose meaning on the world around them."

(Dressler, 2001, p. 455)

Moving beyond family-level dysfunction to include the influence of the surrounding neighborhood and community-level stressors, the aim of the expanded ACE study was to provide a more comprehensive representation of adversity and the effects on health outcomes (Cronholm et al., 2015; Wade et al., 2016). Importantly, the Kaiser-CDC ACEs research included a sample of insured, predominantly white, educated participants and with recognition of socio-structural forces that impact adversity and health outcomes and, given the present-day understanding of health disparities, it can be posited that other unmeasured ACEs also can impact health outcomes, especially in marginalized populations (Cronholm et al., 2015).

Finkelhor, Shattuck, Turner, & Hamby (2013) and Wade et al. (2016) are two investigators who set out to use diverse socio-demographic samples, adding neighborhood and community-level adverse exposures judged by many developmental researchers to be important in predicting long-term health and well-being outcomes. Investigators found that the

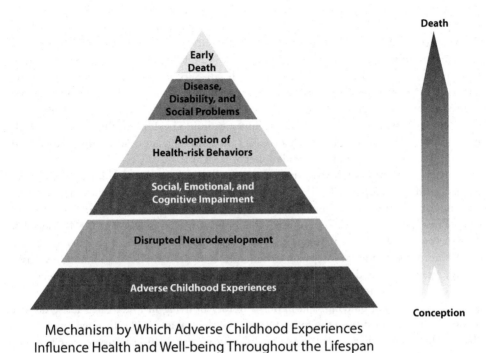

Mechanism by Which Adverse Childhood Experiences
Influence Health and Well-being Throughout the Lifespan

FIGURE 2.1 The ACE Pyramid (CDC, 2016)

association between ACEs and child health was strengthened when exposures such as community violence, property victimization, or bullying were added to the initial ACE index (Finkelhor et al., 2013). Other predictors missing from the ACE Study model include peer rejection, low socioeconomic status, experiencing racism, living in an unsafe neighborhood and having a history with foster care (Cronholm et al., 2015; Wade et al., 2014). Finkelhor et al., (2013) provided data on outcomes incorporating predictors where major childhood adversities are not currently measured by the conventional ACE scale including:

a   *poverty*—longitudinal studies demonstrate that growing up in poverty heightens
    lifetime risk for both a variety of negative life events and health outcomes;
b   *peer rejection*—rejection by friends is linked with the development of many
    disorders (e.g., aggression, poor school competence and psychological maladjustment)
    including overall life status adjustment;
c   *poor school performance*—substandard academic performance during childhood is
    related to poor outcomes in adulthood (e.g., unemployment); and
d   *community violence*—witnessing community violence is linked with mental health
    threat for adults and children.

As an example, within Philadelphia an expanded ACE survey was performed subsequent to the Philadelphia Health Management Corporation's 2012 Southeastern Pennsylvania Household Health Survey (Cronholm et al., 2015). The Household Health Survey, a major comprehensive health survey, used a representative sample of 413,000 child and adult inhabitants from Southeastern Pennsylvania. Employment of a random-digit dialing of land and cell phones was utilized to amass information on a broad range of health matters, conditions, and behaviors. The Philadelphia expanded ACEs survey occurred via phone interview between November 2012 and January 2013 and 1,784 Philadelphia residents over 18 years of age who took part in the original Household Health Survey were recontacted. Interviews conducted by a representative of a survey research firm took an estimated 12 minutes and occurred in both English and Spanish (Cronholm et al., 2015). Of note, interviewers were gender matched with interviewees for this investigation. The Philadelphia expanded ACE survey was designed by the Philadelphia ACEs Task Force, a team of local experts organized by the Institute for Safe Families (Cronholm et al., 2015).

This team was commissioned to study ACEs in Philadelphia. Survey domains that were included in the expanded ACE survey were categorized based on a review of the literature, including data captured from Philadelphia youth regarding community stressors (Wade et al., 2014). That said, parental divorce during childhood was not assessed on the Philadelphia ACEs survey since local data indicated that the construct lacks accurate representation of the complexities of partnered and separated relationships in the sampled communities. Consequently, categories included in expanded ACEs comprised categories beyond conventional ACE categories, such as experiencing racism, witnessing violence, living in an unsafe neighborhood, experiencing bullying, and having a history of living in foster care. These distinct questions were amended from the following surveys: the California Health Interview Survey, Adverse Childhood Experiences International Questionnaire, National Survey on Children's Exposure to Violence, CDC's Family Health History and Health Appraisal Questionnaire, and Perceptions of Racism in Children and Youth instrument (Cronholm et al., 2015; Wade et al., 2016).

Of 1,784 respondents, demographics showed Philadelphia adults were between 18–97 years of age (mean 48.6 years), mainly females (58.3%), race (White, 45.2%; Black, 43.6%), employed (87.8%), single (56.8%), insured (87.7%), and declared a usual source of health care (89.6%) (Cronholm et al., 2015). Furthermore, most respondents earned at least a high school education (89.7%) and household income grossed was above the federal poverty level (69.9%) (Cronholm et al., 2015). When we examine outcomes across all respondents, approximately 20% endorsed four or more conventional ACEs while 10% endorsed three or more expanded ACEs. At least 72.9% of respondents had one conventional ACE and 63.4% had at least one expanded ACE, and when accounting for both 49.3% were affected by one from each category. Interestingly, if only conventional ACEs were used with this sample, 13.9% would have gone unrecognized since this percentage was only affected by expanded ACEs (Cronholm et al., 2015).

Resembling the earlier Kaiser ACE Study, conventional ACE outcomes in this study also resulted in a dose–response relationship on their ACE scores and smoking status, sexually transmitted infections, substance abuse problems, mental health concerns, cardiovascular disease, and fractures (Wade et al., 2016). Contrary to Felitti et al. (1998), there lacked any significant correlation between conventional ACE scores and obesity or diabetes. Notably, expanded ACE scores were significantly correlated with health risk behaviors and mental health concerns; however no significant correlations were linked with physical health conditions. In particular, expanded ACEs revealed a dose–response relationship with sexually transmitted infections and depression but no dose–response relationship with health risk behaviors and poor mental health like conventional ACEs (Wade et al., 2016). Low SES and high ACE scores increased risk for poor mental health as well as substance abuse (Wade et al.,

2016). When examining each expanded ACE indicator for the 1,784 respondents, results showed the following: (a) witnessed violence (40.5%), (b) felt discrimination (34.5%), adverse neighborhood experience (27.3%), being bullied (7.9%), and lived in foster care (2.5%). A comparison of the conventional ACE outcomes between the original study participants and the Philadelphia respondents' are shown in Table 2.1:

TABLE 2.1 Conventional ACE Percentages and Philadelphia ACE Percentages

Abuse	Conventional Study	Philadelphia Study
Emotional—recurrent humiliation	▪ 11%	▪ 33.2%
Physical—beating, not spanking	▪ 28%	▪ 38.1%
Contact sexual abuse	▪ 22%	▪ 16.2%
Neglect		
Physical	▪ 10%	▪ 7%
Emotional	▪ 15%	▪ 7.7%
Household dysfunction		
Mother treated violently	▪ 13%	▪ 20.2%
Household member was alcoholic or drug user	▪ 27%	▪ 34.8%
Household member was imprisoned	▪ 6%	▪ 2.9%
Household member was chronically depressed, suicidal, mentally ill, in psychiatric hospital	▪ 17%	▪ 24.1%
Not raised by both biological parents	▪ 23%	▪ Not/Applicable

ACEs contribute to many adverse health outcomes; however organizations (private, public, government) can leverage their resources to potentially break down barriers in order to eradicate them. As many organizations within the community serve to tackle the social determinants of health, considering wellness from the lens of individual, family, and community within their structural realities is important. By including expanded ACEs into investigations, we capture their effects and this can help support efforts to ameliorate these conditions. Striving to improve the health of socially and economically disenfranchised populations also promotes overall population health. The health care system and health professionals in the United States often attend to health concerns through a focus on individual behavior, genetics, and physiological ailments. It is important for health professionals to consider the larger socio-structural forces (e.g., forces beyond individual and interpersonal interactions) in the lives of individuals that affect health and well-being and the ability to attain health equity. These upstream social and structural factors (e.g., expanded ACEs) must be taken into account when conceptualizing how individuals in the health professions can optimize health care. Health professionals' use of a socio-structural competency frame of reference helps them to more effectively understand their clients' lives in context, and to take action that will have impact on both their physical health and structural conditions (Thompson-Lastad et al., 2017).

3

TOXIC STRESS, ADVERSITY, AND TRAUMA

Toxic stress

Everyone experiences some level of adversity or stress during their lifetime. The stress response represents the physiological and behavioral reaction to discriminating demands from the physical and social environment. Researchers describe toxic stress as the body's sustained exposure to extremely high levels of stress hormones that become damaging, especially during child and adolescent development (Blitz, Anderson, & Saastamoinen, 2016; Shonkoff et al., 2012), promoting health and mental health disparities. These disparities emerge quickly, as 20.5% of children from families living in or approaching poverty display behavioral or emotional problems, compared to 6.4 % of children from economically secure households (Blitz et al., 2016). These demands challenge and disrupt homeostasis responsible for self-regulating the human body to maintain internal stability (Purewal et al., 2016). Because of the undesirable effects of toxic stress, negative attachments frequently signify that children will fall behind in important ways. Consequently, individuals affected by toxic stress endure lifelong hardship, which can cause complications with self-regulation (e.g., defiance, inattention, and impulsivity), learning, executive function, and memory (Walsh & Theodorakakis, 2017). Toxic stress can also heighten one's proneness to physical ailments including cardiovascular disease, obesity, stroke, hypertension, and diabetes as well as mental health difficulties including depression, anxiety disorders, and substance abuse (Walsh & Theodorakakis, 2017). These detrimental effects are reflective of Frederick Douglas's words, "It is easier to build strong children than to repair broken men [and women]" (Goodreads, 2018, p. 1). Many things influence the stress response including a person's perception of the stressor as well as the mental and physical health and genetic composition of the person (Purewal et al., 2016). There is *positive, tolerable, and toxic stress* which is identified on the basis of assumed differences in their likelihood to produce lasting physiologic disruptions due to the intensity and duration of the response (Shonkoff et al., 2012).

Positive stress produces a physiologic condition that is short-lived and mild to moderate in level (e.g., wedding, having a baby, planning a vacation). Fundamentally, key to positive stress, especially for children, is the availability of a compassionate and responsive adult who assists the child to deal with the stressor. This contributes to a protective effect that enables the restoration of the stress response systems to return to baseline status. This experience provides vital opportunities to witness, learn, and practice healthy, adaptive responses to adverse experiences and serve as a growth-promoting element of normal development. *Tolerable stress* involves stressful major life events; nonnormative experiences that pose a great magnitude of adversity or threat. Factors causing these experiences might include the death of a family member, a life-threatening illness or injury, a litigious divorce, a natural disaster, or an act of terrorism (Shonkoff et al., 2012). For a child, when tolerable stress is experienced in the context of a supportive adult who serves as a buffering protection, the risk that such conditions will produce undue activation of the stress response systems that precedes physiologic harm and long-term outcomes for health and learning is significantly diminished (Shonkoff et al., 2012). Accordingly, the fundamental attribute that allows this type of stress response to be tolerable is the level of protective adult relationships that enable the child's adaptive coping and a feeling of control.

Toxic Stress, a term coined by the Harvard University Center on the Developing Child, is the most dangerous type of stress response. Toxic stress ensues from intense, frequent, and/or prolonged activation of the body's stress response and autonomic nervous system lacking the safeguarding of a caring adult (Dowd, 2017; Purewal et al., 2016). The age when someone is exposed to toxic stress is an important factor to consider; the younger the brain, the more vulnerable it is to the harmful effect of toxic stress (Dowd, 2017). Analogous to other ecological toxins such as heavy metals, social and emotional toxic stress causes epigenetic variations that influence how genes show up or are suppressed via processes, for example, DNA methylation and histone alteration memory (Walsh & Theodorakakis, 2017). Because of chronic dysregulation of the neuro-endocrine immune network caused by chronic stress, the body is not able to return to homeostasis (Blitz et al., 2016). When there is chronic dysregulation of the neuro-endocrine immune network early in life resulting from ACEs, activation of the stress response becomes toxic in contexts that are non-nurturing for the child or if the child has biological or genetic vulnerabilities to stress (Shonkoff et al., 2012). Although a stress response is adaptive when responding to instant, acute danger (i.e., flight or fight response), experiencing toxic stress can cause persistent activation of the stress response and consequentially exposure to stress hormones (Blanch, Shern, & Steverman, 2014). This chronic activation disrupts brain circuitry and other organ and metabolic systems during sensitive developmental periods (i.e. points in maturation when environmental input has the greatest influence on development) triggering a dysregulation of the stress response system, known as biological embedding of experience (Anderson, 2015). This disruption can produce anatomic changes and/or physiologic dysregulations. Importantly, these are the antecedents of later deficiencies in learning and behavior along with being the bases of persistent, stress-related physical and behavioral health concerns (Blanch et al., 2014). The role toxic stress plays in early life adversity and in the pathological process of health disparities draws attention to the importance of effective examination for substantive risk factors in the health care setting, especially primary care. Furthermore, there is a need for students in the health professions and practicing health professionals to move past the level of risk factor recognition. Leveraging innovations in the biology of adversity is required to further the essential undertaking of developing, assessing, and enhancing novel and more effective approaches to decreasing toxic stress and alleviating its effects earlier, before irreversible harm occurs (Blanch et al., 2014).

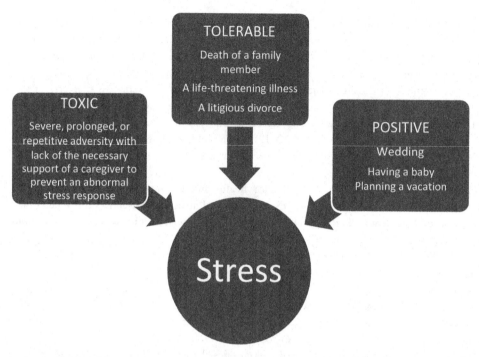

FIGURE 3.1 Types of Stress

Adversity

Adversity, a state, condition, or occurrence of critical or prolonged difficulty, consists of dele-terious life conditions acknowledged to be significantly related to adjustment problems that can have an effect on a person's development, mental and physical health, as well as learning (Bloom, 2013). These adjustment concerns can range in severity and duration. Also, each adversity is distinctive, customarily produced by numerous causes. Therefore, an individual's response to adversity in their environment will differ as a function of personal dispositions, socialization practices, the form and timing of the adversity, and the counteracting supports accessible to them in their respective environments (Osher et al., 2017). Obviously, the term adversity is applied to indicate experiences that are challenging and have a negative implication.

For youth, exposure to adversity and stressors including poverty, lack of safety and stability in the family environment, and lack of access to quality early education can unfavorably affect their development. Kuras and colleagues (2017) highlight that early life adversity involves many negative experiences preceding adulthood, ranging from unpleasant to traumatic, with exam-ples including physical, emotional, or sexual abuse, neglect, separation from parent, parental loss, instances of domestic or community violence, or natural disaster. These adversities consist of experiences that are liable to require significant adaptation by an average child and that characterize a divergence from the expected environment (McLaughlin, 2016). These expo-sures can lead to an at-risk or vulnerable course in life and in serious instances a delayed or chaotic life course prevails. Moreover, it is estimated that up to 50% of the population is exposed to adversity during the course of development (Anderson, 2015; McLaughlin, 2016). Similarly, the World Health Organization approximates that, across countries with broadly

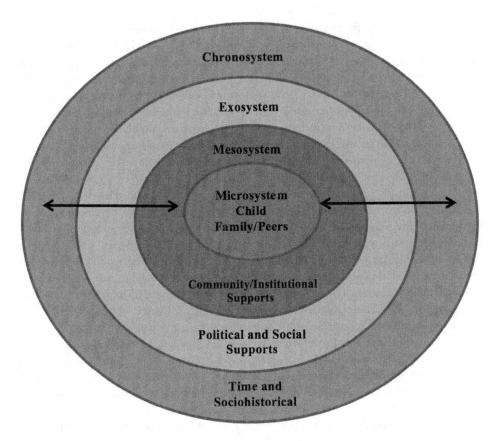

FIGURE 3.2 Adversity Diagram

variable levels of economic development, about 40% of children experience at least one adverse event. Interestingly, of those 40%, children have a 60% chance of experiencing a second adverse event (Kuras et al., 2017). Adverse experiences frequently co-occur, especially among disadvantaged populations, yet they are frequently investigated in isolation; adverse experiences also tend to persist over time (Ramos–Olazagasti, Bird, Canino, & Duarte, 2017).

The lens used to examine adversity is important to consider. Individual, ecological, as well as cultural and contextual factors are key areas to reflect on. Individually, the level or severity of hardship a person encounters can enhance their vulnerability depending on factors such as personality traits, adaptive coping strategies implemented, and age. For example, a person encountering severe adversity with limited adaptive coping is more likely to experience post-traumatic stress disorder (PTSD) which poses a significant threat to their well-being (Ungar, 2015). Similarly, when stressors occur at one or more systemic levels (micro-meso-exo-chrono systems), interactions between factors at different levels occur. Peering through an ecological lens, fetal alcohol spectrum disorder, family violence, and only having access to a poorly resourced school may encumber a child more than less complex adversity that involves a single system (e.g. a child who displays signs of PTSD after a sexual assault is apt to recover faster when they are well-supported both psychologically and physically) (Ungar, 2015). Importantly, potential vulnerability and the capability to overcome hardship may be viewed as comprising numerous biological, psychological, and social systems and their interactions (Ungar, 2015).

A person's biosystem, for instance, consists of interactions that either hinder or augment neurological functioning and gene expression (Ungar, 2015). Additionally, the human body is a bioecological microsystem wherein physical subsystems are affected by cognitive and emotional processes. The bioecological model of development postulates that children develop through interactions with individuals, groups and structures within their proximal and distal contexts. Developmental perspectives pertaining to the bioecological theory extend outward from the micro level to include mesosystems, or interactions between microsystems; exosystems, or exchanges between microsystems and larger systems; as well as macrosystems, or larger social or cultural contexts wherein an individual's development occurs (Olofson, 2017). As an illustration, microsystemic interactions relate to those between children and their social groups (e.g., school classmates or caregivers) or could be related to the family environment which influences development by shaping the cognitive development of the child through the support and the conflict that is present in the home (Olofson, 2017). Exemplification of mesosystemic interactions, when microsystems interact, could be those between a foster child's social service workers, teachers, and behavioral health care providers. Each of these develop their own microsystems which can assist a child to manage better with an out-of-home placement (Ungar, 2015). Mesosystemic interactions impact the likelihood that individuals can acquire social supports; therefore, the quality of the mesosystem is extremely important to adjustment and positive development when adversity emerges in a person's life, which has a major influence on the development of psychological resilience (Olofson, 2017). Representation of exosystemic social processes can include social policies, neighbors, legal services, court systems, social welfare services, mass media, as well as friends and family. The exosystem involves the interconnectedness between the micro-and meso-systems and those systems wherein the individual has no direct contact, but can affect the functioning of these two systems. Lastly, chronosystems describe patterning of environmental outcomes along with transitions over the life course including the sociohistorical period in which adjustments to stress/adversity transpire (Williams, 2016). An important assumption of taking a micro-meso-exo-chrono systemic perspective is that early inequities that heighten a person's exposure to stress are prone to accumulate over time, changing from prolonged stress and precarious behaviors into chronic and serious diseases. This perspective is modeled after the concept of allostatic load. This refers to "wear and tear" that occurs throughout the life course or, to be more exact, the cumulative physiologic toll taken on the body during the lifetime of attempts a person takes to acclimate to life's demands (Osher et al., 2017).

Trauma

Trauma, "an emotional and physical response that occurs when a person's internal and external resources are inadequate to cope with an external threat," stems from the Greek term for wound (τραῦμα) related to physical injury (Danese & Baldwin, 2017; Feuer-Edwards, O'Brien, & O'Connor, 2016, p. 8). However, during the 19th century, the term trauma began to obtain a new emblematic connotation in popular culture. It was during the Industrial Revolution that Victorian surgeons became mystified by psychological and physical symptoms emerging in those wounded by railway accidents but lacked obvious physical wounds (Danese & Baldwin, 2017). German neurologist Hermann Oppenheim proposed that symptoms were produced by imperceptible physical injury to the spine or brain (Danese & Baldwin, 2017). Interestingly, there was a high prevalence of histories of childhood abuse

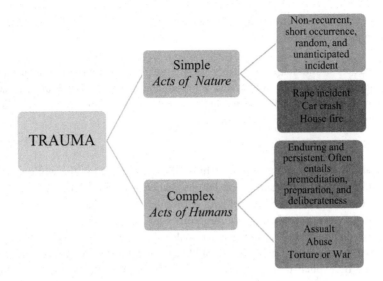

FIGURE 3.3 Types of Trauma

observed among individuals with inexplicable somatic and emotional conditions, and prominent French neurologists Jean-Martin Charcot and Pierre Janet hypothesized that the symptoms were triggered by trauma (Danese & Baldwin, 2017) They saw trauma as the subjective view of powerfully distressing experiences which elicit psychological and physical symptoms (hysteria) (Danese & Baldwin, 2017). Of note, Sigmund Freud, an Austrian psychiatrist, extended Charcot and Janet's psychological theory and spread the idea that powerfully upsetting experiences (i.e., psychological traumas, especially those taking place in childhood) may well have substantial effects on both psychological development and psychopathology (Danese & Baldwin, 2017).

In Greyber and colleagues (2015), the Child Trauma Academy asserts that trauma is a "psychologically distressing event that is outside the range of usual human experience, one that induces an abnormally intense and prolonged stress response" (p. 188). Likewise, trauma is referred to as

> a reaction to a kind of wound. It is a reaction to profoundly injurious events and situations in the real world and, indeed, to a world in which people are routinely wounded and thus, traumatizing socio-political circumstances must be part of the understanding and addressing of people's psychosocial problems.
>
> *(Quiros & Berger, 2015, p. 4)*

The latter definition is rare since often there is a failure to attend to socio-political experiences leading to a rigid understanding and conceptualization of trauma. Andermahr (2015) poses a similar concern stating that a chief stumbling block is that trauma theory persists with following the traditional event-based model of trauma; consequently, trauma is perceived to arise from a single, extraordinary, disastrous event. Frequently, trauma is described as an alarming event outside of normal experience; however this typical model of trauma lacks authenticity for non-Western and/or minority group trauma including populations within

Western societies (Andermahr, 2015). Specifically, the experience of racism is not recognized if using the typical forms of trauma:

> Unlike structural trauma, racism is historically specific; yet, unlike historical trauma, it is not related to a particular event, with a before and an after. Understanding racism as a historical trauma, which can be worked through, would be to obscure the fact that it continues to cause damage in the present.
>
> *(Andermahr, 2015, p. 2)*

As a result, racially-based systems of trauma historically entrenched in the worldwide practices of slavery and colonialism present a momentous challenge to the Eurocentric representation of trauma as a single overwhelming incident. Moreover, recognizing racism as trauma within a racialized society poses a dilemma in numerous ways; specifically, it can subsist in a concealed manner, its consequences are generational, and its consequences can be ascribed to other causes, all of which profit from and uphold its obscured nature. In this structure, racism is not sustained by explicit prejudice; however it is clandestine and ostensibly unintended to those for whom the system advantages and is flagrant and agonizing to those for whom it is not. There is a blatant distinction between persons who have the privilege of disregarding the origin of the present-day order of things, nevertheless realize all the advantages, and people who do not and cannot. Ignoring these facts is not only a location of privilege but an operational need for upholding the status quo of increasing success, security, and provision—this is completely at the expense of others' lives. Neglecting these truths, then, is not insignificant; it is a calamity. Individuals existing within the other non-dominant sphere bear the effects and wounds of the history in their actual bodies, shouldering the burden of it every day. This is an experience of trauma (Greer, 2017).

By decolonizing trauma, an account of the particular social and historical settings in which narratives regarding trauma are constructed and received is recognized, along with being open and attentive to the varied strategies of representation and opposition that these settings invite or necessitate (Andermahr, 2015). If the ethical aspirations of health professionals is to be realized, as we examine trauma-related research we must decolonize trauma studies and distinguish the globalized circumstances of traumatic events, the particular forms traumatic suffering takes, and the numerous ways in which it is characterized in scholarly compositions. Understanding decolonized trauma in this way would be beneficial: (a) as reparation to the marginalization of non-Western and minority traumas; (b) as a challenge to the assumed universal authority of Western characterizations of trauma; (c) affording choices to prevailing trauma aesthetics; and (d) attending to the underexplored association between professed First and Third World traumas (Andermahr, 2015). Privileging the understanding of interpersonal trauma over sociopolitical trauma typically occurs in today's society though harmful effects of historical socio-political stressors have been supported. This is directly related to who is in power and whose voice supersedes in defining trauma. Determination of traumatic experiences relies on the subjective interpretation of the events not objective reality so we must know whose subjective reality is being represented in our understanding of trauma, treatment protocols, diagnostic categorization, and other policy-related decisions (Quiros & Berger, 2015).

When trauma occurs is quite important. While trauma may be experienced at any point in one's life, research indicates that when troublesome events are experienced in childhood, they can produce significant impairments to social, emotional, and cognitive development

(Feuer-Edwards et al., 2016). Also, though traumatic events occurring in childhood represent one potential form of childhood adversity, not all types of childhood adversity are traumatic. According to McLaughlin (2016), examples of adverse childhood experiences that may not be considered traumatic are neglect; poverty; and the absence of a stable, supportive caregiver; of note, this perspective is based on traditional protocol used in psychiatry. Interestingly, child and adolescent populations have similar distributions as it relates to traumatic experience; an estimated 48 % of children abused are male and 52 % are female (Greyber et al., 2015). Epidemiological examination suggests that between 58%–90% of youths have experienced a minimum of one trauma, with most trauma survivors experiencing numerous traumatic events (Martin et al., 2016). Each person's response to trauma will vary subject to their history of trauma, quality and quantity of social support, levels of resilience, and temperament (Feuer-Edwards et al., 2016). Furthermore, the effects of a traumatic experience vary based on the magnitude of its impact; though often trauma resolves by itself, in other instances the traumatic response remains hidden up until the person is activated (Feuer-Edwards et al., 2016). Additionally, post-traumatic stress could impact others; as such, people will experience extreme levels of stress for a number of days or weeks subsequent to a significant event. If not properly attended to post-traumatic stress can produce Post-Traumatic Stress Disorder with symptoms exhibited for at least three months after the event (Feuer-Edwards et al., 2016). Of note, trauma is a devastating experience that can demoralize a person's belief in the goodness and safety of the world.

During childhood, traumatization arises when he/she observes an external threat; and subsequently suffers an acute distress signal reaction that activates the body's stress response with enduring impairment to vital neurological and psychological systems (Brunzell, Stokes, & Waters, 2016). When infants and children encounter trauma, the developing brain is adversely affected along with healthy attachment to the primary person taking care of the infant/child (Brunzell et al., 2016). Essentially, trauma impacts all aspects of youths' development. However, from a neurodevelopmental standpoint, trauma is not an event; it is viewed from the person's response to the incident and enduring effects on the varied stress-related physiological systems (e.g., the autonomic, neuroimmune, neuroendocrine, central nervous system) (Brunzell et al., 2016). Traumatic events produce extreme feelings of fear, helplessness, hopelessness, hypervigilance, shame, guilt, anger, isolation, and detachment; as well, interpersonal relationships can be marred.

Traumatic incidents are frequently referred to as type one (i.e., simple trauma, acute trauma, or acts of God) and type two (complex trauma or acts of humans) (Brunzell et al., 2016; Courtois & Gold, 2009). Type one trauma, which we will refer to as acts of nature, acute trauma, is distinguished as a non-recurrent, short occurrence, random, and unanticipated incident such as a lone rape incident, car crash, house fire, or a natural disaster. The experience of a simple traumatic incident may be life threatening or may imminently bring about serious harm. Oftentimes, there is diminished stigma and blame projected towards the victim, and the trauma is frequently tied to a community response regarding the incident (Brunzell et al., 2016; Greyber et al., 2015).

On the contrary, type two trauma (i.e., complex trauma, development or relationship trauma) characteristically starts in childhood and is enduring, persistent, and continuous. Type two trauma typically produces long-lasting characterological and relational difficulties and the likelihood increases of being effected by a trauma-related disorder (e.g., dissociative disorders, substance and alcohol use or abuse, as well as PTSD) (Brunzell et al., 2016). Notably, complex trauma is most often human induced; specifically, it is committed by individuals who are part of the caregiving system and consequently produces a huge amount of suffering that habitually continues into adulthood (Courtois & Gold, 2009; Greyber et al., 2015). Most often, incidents of complex trauma entail premeditation, preparation, and deliberateness in their execution. For example, actions that fall into this classification comprise all types of assault (e.g., sexual and physical), abuse (e.g., psychological and verbal), intimidation, acts of violence and torture, war and genocide, as well as human trafficking (Courtois & Gold, 2009). Betrayal-trauma, a markedly potent form of human-induced trauma, occurs when people or institutions perpetuate these acts on an individual who is dependent. Intrinsically, betrayal-traumas in children frequently consist of loss of trust that underlies primary caregiving relationships (Edmonds, Hampson, Côté, Hill, & Klest, 2016). More specifically, Courtois and Gold (2009) argue that interpersonal or attachment trauma and all types of domestic violence and child abuse (e.g., physical, emotional and sexual including incest), and neglect committed by related and trusted individuals within and outside of the family, comprise betrayal-trauma. Additional types of betrayal-trauma are located in institutions where abuse of certain members by others (e.g., sexual harassment or sexual assault) is clandestinely permitted although visibly prohibited, and is poorly responded to when reported (Courtois & Gold, 2009). More egregiously is when the victim is criticized for its incidence and for complaining about the betrayal. Because betrayal-trauma underscores the relational context within which trauma occurs, when physical abuse and sexual abuse is committed by caregivers these are seen as more highly significant betrayals than are oppressive persecutory acts executed by strangers or individuals in circumstances whereby trust or dependence on the perpetrator for physical or emotional needs is nonexistent (Martin, Van Ryzin, & Dishion, 2016). When equated with other forms of trauma, those including greater levels of betrayal have routinely been linked with more symptom severity across numerous mental health outcomes, involving depression, PTSD, anxiety, as well as hallucinations (Martin et al., 2016).

How society and more specifically health professionals define and perceive trauma must be examined. Bloom (2013) and Rich et al. (2009) state that history encourages us to not only be mindful of how trauma is defined, but also who is included in defining trauma and the effects on victims or survivors, even when there is evident change occurring related to societal awareness (Bloom, 2013). For health professionals, if a core ethical principle of your professional practice is to promote social justice, structural and environmental conditions must be taken into account when assessing trauma, challenging traditional psychiatry and diagnostic categorization. More specifically, conceptualization, understanding, assessment and diagnosis of trauma must extend beyond the micro-level to consider social conditions and political factors that augment trauma in the lives of people. By incorporating intersectionality of race, class and gender and other cultural factors among oppressed groups, inclusivity in understanding trauma occurs (Rich et al., 2009). It affords credence to how people's socio-cultural location interacts with the other above-mentioned systems of power and oppression to regulate making meaning of their lived experiences. What's more, absent from the definition of traumatic experiences is systemic oppression; this is because the wounded are characteristically oppressed groups whose voices are shut down by the universality of society's normed population (i.e., white, middle-class and heterosexual experiences that govern the treatment and research literature) (Quiros & Berger, 2015).

Trauma is inseparable from systems of power and oppression (Becker-Blease, 2017). Too often, society is appalled with trauma survivors, particularly symptoms they display and the burdens our social system must absorb from health care, child welfare, judicial, and educational systems. It is quite unfortunate that society at large is not horrified and disgusted by the systems of oppression that cause such trauma for these victims. For example, when an individual seeks help after being sexually assaulted at work, responses are accompanied by rejection, criticism, questioning, or maltreatment/substandard care (i.e., administrative, medical or psychological treatment) (Courtois & Gold, 2009). Similar responses can occur in cultural and ethnic groups where stringent punishments are employed by the family or a larger community if a person functions outside of imposed norms (i.e., honor killings or genital mutilation/ female circumcision) (Courtois & Gold, 2009).

In closing, while trauma may have dissimilar meanings across cultures, no population is exempt from experiencing trauma. Moreover, the repercussions of trauma are not equally distributed in society (Bowen & Murshid, 2016). Younger populations are most vulnerable and notably some forms of trauma are unduly experienced by particular populations due to profoundly rooted structural inequalities aligned with sources of power. Individuals with limited resources, especially those living in poverty and racial minorities in the United States experience disproportionate trauma at the individual, family and community level. Health professionals' understanding about the unequal structuring of trauma across different segments of society and the narrow medicalized focus often implemented, must be attended to in order to mitigate the wounds/suffering endured by our fellow man due to structured processes and forces (social, economic and political) that are normed within our society.

Taking conventional ACEs to another level requires deepened understanding about toxic stress, adversity and trauma and consequent health outcomes integrating insights crossing disciplinary sciences, intervening professionals, structural competency and sociopolitical realms. Health professionals working with these populations across the life course and attending to the inclusive lived experiences of their clientele, are critical advocates given the wide-ranging domains of employment in which they practice.

PART II

Understanding ACEs from a life course health development perspective

4

THE BODY KEEPS THE SCORE

Epigenetics

Many individuals will confront some form of trauma or severe stress during their lifetime; however, most have the ability to recuperate from such events without any long-term health consequences. Some individuals are more vulnerable to stress and trauma, along with the physical and mental health effects after such an exposure. Varying levels of vulnerability are potentially influenced by genetic susceptibility and particular characteristics of the stress itself (e.g., nature, intensity and duration), in addition to epigenetic mechanisms. Epigenetics is concerned with how environmental exposures and experiences inform gene expression (Brendtro, 2015). Loi, Del Savio, and Stupka (2013) assert that epigenetics is described as the "study of the inheritance (between cells and/or organisms) of traits (gene expression or phenotypes) without changes to the underlying DNA sequence" (p. 142). The prefix "epi" implies on top of or over the genome; there is no alteration of the inherited genomic structure itself. Therefore, this indicates why genes alone do not determine a person's fate; essentially epigenetics pertaining to human beings suggests that which controls the person beyond genetics. While epigenetics is not genetics; epigenetics can defy genetics (Brendtro, 2015). Changes in gene expression created by experience means that new experiences may create new changes (Brendtro & Mitchell, 2014). In fact, life experiences encountered in the environment actually turn genes on or off (Brendtro, 2015). Importantly, we now know that lifelong differences in gene function may well be caused by processes other than gene sequence variations—epigenetic processes (Szyf & Meaney, 2008). These processes can uniquely mediate the enduring impact of social environmental exposure and fetal development (Szyf & Meaney, 2008). The resilient human brain has remarkable neuroplasticity and is able to redesign itself well into maturity. Advancements in learnings about epigenetics have promoted understanding more fully how a person's health is affected by early developmental events and previous generations' environmental circumstances (Loi et al., 2013). This chapter reflects van der Kolk's perspective when he stated, "What you can't see, can hurt you! (Brous, 2014, p.1).

Human beings have more than 20,000 genes, and most of them influence the brain. Brendtro (2015) stated that all genes are in practically every bodily cell; nevertheless, only those turned on (i.e., expressed) communicate to the cell what it is supposed to do. In 2012, the ENCODE Project Consortium avowed that three million gene controls actually control this gene expression (Brendtro, 2015). For example, unremitting long-term stress, chemicals, nutritional regime, and caregiving all can produce epigenetic effects. Specific to stress, nurturing care turns on genes in the brain that govern stress, creating children that are social, inquisitive and confident. Conversely, neglect creates stressed, apprehensive children. Since epigenetics is linked to experience, it is therefore theoretically reversible (Brendtro, 2015). Epigenetics is implicated in numerous physical and mental ailments by which the gene-environment interaction gets under the skin, but importantly, healthy environments and cultures create hardy bodies and brains (Brendtro, 2015). Understanding the science of epigenetics has implications for health professionals' ability to understand, prevent, and treat health-related disorders. The dynamism of epigenetic regulation compared to the static nature of the gene sequence offers a process for altering gene function as a result of changes in lifestyle, possibly through behavioral or therapeutic intervention (Szyf & Meaney, 2008).

Epigenetics has rekindled attention to new knowledge regarding the lasting influences social life can have on the body and the possibility that acquired characteristics may well be transmitted from generation to generation (Lappé, 2016). By advancing a link between social life and how genes are expressed, epigenetics proposes a paradigm shift in considering the links between nature and nurture. Instead of beginning life simply with the genes transferred from a person's mother and father, there is awareness that the effect of their experiences and for that matter, that of a person's earlier generations, may indeed be transmitted as well. Accordingly, epigenetics has the ability to generate a more holistic perception of health and can therefore stimulate investment of resources in social and environmental conditions that influence human well-being (Lappé, 2016).

To that end, the next section will address three specific ways epigenetic modification generally happens: (1) through attachment of a methyl group to the back of a DNA molecule, in effect, turning off a transcription of a related gene, (2) through modification of the histones in which the DNA is wrapped, consequently this causes the DNA to unravel and become more accessible to transcription factors, and (3) through microRNA regulation (Lappé, 2016).

Social environment and DNA methylation

Environmental programming of the stress response through alterations in DNA methylation, one of several ways in which the epigenome can influence gene expression is the most studied and best characterized epigenetic mark (Fiori & Turecki, 2016). Given that DNA methylation can change the manner in which genes express themselves without causing alteration in the actual sequence of the genes, nonetheless having functional consequences is momentous (Szyf, Tang, Hill, & Musci, 2016). DNA methylation involves the attachment of a methyl group (consisting of one carbon and three hydrogen atoms) to nucleotides in an individual's DNA which blocks the activation of a gene. The sites where a cytosine nucleotide appears beside a guanine nucleotide (CpG dinucleotides), are believed to be the most stable form of epigenetic alteration (Szyf et al., 2016). Methylation can block the binding of transcription factors or affect gene expression through other processes (Klengel, Pape, Binder, & Mehta, 2014; Yang et al., 2014). Furthermore, genes that are highly expressed characteristically have low levels of promoter methylation (Szyf et al., 2016; Tyrka et al., 2015; Wagner et al., 2014). DNA methylation in gene regulatory regions, such as promoters or enhancers, is frequently linked with gene repression as a result of recruitment of methyl-binding proteins. These proteins produce chromatin condensation or interference with transcription factor binding (Fiori & Turecki, 2016). Likewise, DNA could be silenced depending on its state of methylation. Methylation of critical regulatory areas of genes can silence gene expression by either impeding access to factors that enlist the transcription machinery that transcribes the genes or via recruitment of proteins that alter the chromatin and close the chromatin surrounding the gene (Szyf et al., 2016).

Social environment is important since early adverse life conditions may have greater influence on DNA methylation; this implies the attendance of critical or sensitive periods for the epigenetic impacts of early life adversity (Fiori & Turecki, 2016). For example, childhood adversity was first shown to influence methylation patterns of the glucocorticoid receptor gene (*NR3C1*) in the brain; however it has been implicated in other tissues as well. Mitchell, Schneper, and Notterman (2016) argue that childhood adversity may well cause many epigenetic changes into the thousands of CpG sites.

van IJzendoorn and colleagues (van IJzendoorn, Bakermans-Kranenburg, & Ebstein, 2011) described child development as "experiences being sculpted in the organism's DNA through methylation" (p. 305). These stressful social conditions alter DNA methylation and this may lead to psychological and physical ailments. DNA methylation is increasingly being recognized for its role in mediating gene-environment interplay throughout the lifespan with dynamic changes found in central nervous system DNA methylation during early development and in adulthood (Mitchell et al., 2016). For example, prenatal maternal stress alters placental function. It is likely that these effects are regulated by changes in placental methylation patterns (Mitchell et al., 2016). The enduring consequences of epigenetically moderated placenta dysfunction on health and behavior of a child are undoubtedly moderated by postnatal parenting choices. Therefore, opportunities exist to alter adverse effects that may have occurred earlier. Even more extensive processes of the social environment, including neighborhoods or communities, may have some effect on methylation patterns (Mitchell et al., 2016). This process entails reversibility of DNA myelination.

Szyf and colleagues (2016) contend that if DNA can be methylated then it can be demethylated in response to environmental signals since methylation occurs by responding to experiences that occur in fully differentiated tissue. Similarly, reversibility of DNA methylation is essential when considering interventions intended to reset epigenetic programming. While the processes accountable for demethylation are thus far indistinct, there is confirmation that DNA methylation is potentially reversible in mature, completely differentiated neurons. Realizing this has two vital propositions: (a) DNA methylation may well change in adult tissues; as such, even adult tissue ought to be potentially reactive to environmental signals and modification of phenotypes could hypothetically happen in adults and (b) it should be conceivable to intervene to reverse DNA methylation in mature cells and lessen unfavorable phenotypes (Szyf et al., 2016).

Modification of histones

Epigenetic mechanisms are frequently regulated by posttranslational modifications of chemical changes in histones. Histones, small structural proteins that DNA is wrapped around, make up the basic unit of chromatin which is the nucleosome that permits the DNA to be compactly stored to fit into the nucleus. Importantly, chromatin is the complex of DNA and the associated histone proteins (Lester, Conradt, & Marsit, 2016). Changes in how DNA is wrapped around the histones contribute to changes in gene expression. Histone modification, one central mechanism that enables alteration in chromatin to take effect, is posttranslational; that is, it occurs after the protein is produced, frequently while it is in place at the nucleosome. Posttranslational encompasses numerous ways in which molecules attach to the tails that project from the histones and modify the activity of the DNA wrapped around them. Of note, histone modification is part of molecular memory of adverse early stress and key pathways through which the environment gets under an individual's skin (Drury, Sánchez, & Gonzalez, 2016).

Environmental factors frequently affect chromatin structure via direct interaction with enzymes that alter histone codes. Also, histone modifications strongly influence chromatin structure. Chromatin remodeling involves covalent alterations at the level of histone tails to support an open or closed chromatin structure. To distinguish the two, open chromatin (i.e., euchromatin) relates to the accessibility to transcriptional factors and heightened rates of gene expression. However, closed chromatin structures (i.e., heterochromatin) are associated with repressed transcription and silences gene expression (Dias, Maddox, Klengel, & Ressler, 2015).

Histones which have protruding N- and C-terminal tails that undergo covalent post-translational modifications can be altered by discrete and precise enzymes including methylation, acetylation, phosphorylation, and ubiquitination (Adav et al., 2018). These modifications typically have a major impact on the chromatin higher-order structure and gene transcription. These posttranslational modifications generally affect protein functions or gene expression, eventually affecting biological processes (Adav et al., 2018). Critical roles performed by histones in gene transcription regulation are based on functional capacity categorized into two groups (Adav et al., 2018). One group, histone H1, is identified as the linker histones; these histones close loops of DNA and make nucleosome structures compact and therefore are prone to be repressors of transcription. The second group, histone complexes which are protein octamers with 2 copies each of histone H2A, H2B, H3, and H4 are identified as core histones (Adav et al., 2018). Both the linker and core histones, which have their amino acids exposed to covalent alterations predominantly in the N-terminal tails, are components of histone modifier mechanisms. Consequently, post-translational modifications of histone tails are associated with transcriptionally active or inactive chromatin states.

In general, acetylation of histones H3 and H4 loosens the interaction between DNA and histones and allows the transcriptional mechanism access to the promoters of particular genes. Thus, hyperacetylation at the promoters increases transcriptional activity, whereas hypoacetylation decreases activity; histone acetylation at lysine (K) residues is generally viewed as one of the epigenetic marks related to active chromatin (i.e., euchromatin) (Szyf, 2016). However, high histone methylation, which does not change the overall charge of the nucleosome generally, is linked with more condensed chromatin states and gene repression. Interestingly, methylation is linked with both transcriptional activation and repression and these are dependent on several factors such as the specific histone subunit, residue, and methylation state. For example, H3K4 methylation is considered as a gene activation signal, whereas H3K9 and H3K27 methylation is correlated with transcription repression (Lo & Zhou, 2014). Both DNA methylation and histone modifications commonly act synergistically to regulate gene expression (Dias et al., 2015). Importantly, histone acetylation is a reversible development; the enzymes that catalyze the reversal of histone acetylation are identified as histone deacetylases.

Pointedly, early life stress and adversity modifies the epigenome by numerous mechanisms with effects persisting into adulthood. Stress also regulates gene expression through bi-directional changes in histone acetylation among other factors. The behavioral neuroscience discipline identifies that posttranslational histone modification occurs at memory-linked gene promoters to alter chromatin structure and subsequently control transcription of the genes in response to environmental cues. For example, histone protein modifications in brain tissue in response to stress occur rapidly; therefore, changes associated with stress-reducing practices like mindfulness-based treatment may be likewise fast acting (Niles, Mehta, Corrigan, Bhasin, & Denninger, 2014). Specifically, selective downregulation of histone deacetylase genes (i.e., HDAC2, HDAC3, and HDAC9) has been detected after a single eight-hour meditation refuge. This indicates the probability of prompt epigenetic activity after mindfulness-based treatment (Niles et al., 2014). Accordingly, epigenetics has challenged the dichotomy between "nature and nurture" because the epigenome can be viewed as a molecular interface between the environment and the genome that is influenced by genetic sequence but constantly receives regulatory feedback by environmental cues (e.g., early life stress, ACEs) and can shape gene function and behavioral response to the environment.

Micro RNA regulation

MicroRNAs (miRNAs), another form of epigenetic regulation, are small non-coding RNAs that are typically 20 to 30 nucleotides in length (Barchitta, Maugeri, Quattrocchi, Agrifoglio, & Agodi, 2017). miRNAs cause gene silencing post-transcriptionally by either suppressing translation or inducing degradation of mRNA (Barchitta et al., 2017; Blaze, Asok, & Roth, 2015). As endogenous, short, noncoding molecules, miRNA can regulate the expression of several genes, while one gene can be targeted by different miRNAs. Thus, miRNAs can regulate up to 60% of our genome, and each miRNA likely modulates the expression of 200 target genes (Hollins & Cairns, 2016; Osborne-Majnik, Fu, & Lane, 2013). In effect, miRNAs characterize essential epigenetic processes of regulation that can control complex processes including cell growth, differentiation, stress response, and tissue remodelling, thus potentially performing a crucial role in many disease states (Barchitta et al., 2017). Andolina, di Segni, and Ventura (2017) argue that thanks to miRNAs' ability to modify gene expression, they can influence gene expression patterns promoting an organism's adaptation to internal and environmental or external factors including stressful events.

Importantly, miRNAs are abundant in the human brain and they have the ability to modulate the neuronal and cellular stress response. miRNAs and their widespread gene networks afford a process to both propel essential developmental initiatives and uphold system homeostasis which is important at times of environmental adversity. These processes may be modifying the system dynamics to deliver the most suitable conditions to safeguard against cellular crisis (Hollins & Cairns, 2016). The instigation of the stress response by the central nervous system is needed to maintain health and homeostasis, nevertheless, there are also effects as these processes can stimulate important changes in neural structure and function that lead to the development of a broad range of psychopathology (Hollins & Cairns, 2016). Stressors may be physiological, including exposure to contaminants or nutrient deficiency or they can be psychological, happening when an individual is confronted with a situation believed to surpass their potential for coping. These stressors create physiological and psychological responses (e.g., high blood pressure, elevated corticosteroids and deficits in sustained attention) (Hollins & Cairns, 2016). Importantly, exposure to environmental stressors can generate changes in manifestation of genes implicated in the modulation of miRNA expression, in addition to alterations in expression of miRNA concerned with the development and function of the central nervous system (Hollins & Cairns, 2016).

miRNAs are associated with neuroplasticity and stress-related disorders such as anxiety, depression, and bipolar disorder. Also, early life stress contributes to increased manifestation of varied miRNAs in the prefrontal cortex (Aschrafi et al., 2016). When stressful circumstances take place, miRNAs are ideally situated to enhance stress responses via dynamic modulation of gene expression through quick and reversible responses. Still, regulation of the stress response necessitates an intensive effort by many miRNA, consisting of miRNA clusters and families. While miRNAs are initially a protective mechanism, stress-induced modifications in miRNA expression are connected to neurodegeneration and the pathogenesis of neurodegenerative diseases (Hollins & Cairns, 2016). Andolina and colleagues' (2017) research identifies that members of the miRNA-34 family of miRNAs are vital modulators of stress response with their function in the expression of fear and anxiety-related behaviors. Intriguingly, miRNA 34c is believed to be up-regulated in the central nucleus of the amygdala after acute and chronic stress. Furthermore, local inhibition of miRNA-34c is thought to increase anxiety-like behavior (Andolina et al., 2017). Regarding the stress response, Aschrafi et al. (2016) also denote that acute stress modifies other members of the miRNA family; specifically, miR-183 and miR-134 levels in the amygdala. However, miR-144 and miR-16 levels are modified in the blood in a naturalistic stress situation, for instance when taking an academic examination (Aschrafi et al., 2016). Interestingly, there is an observed decline met during aging in stress attenuation. Specifically, the strength of the response to stress is reduced as age increases. Consequently, the expression of miRNA requires balance to not exceed threshold levels, to avoid stress attenuation (Hollins & Cairns, 2016).

Taken together, when confronted with stress a cascade of psychophysiological responses are mobilized, even though adaptive coping and post-stress recovery is mainly contingent on optimal neuronal functioning which necessitates specific and rapid gene expression changes (Vaisvaser et al., 2016). This may be accomplished via post-transcriptional regulation through miRNAs recognizing that each miRNA can target up to hundreds of genes, generally regulating about half of the transcriptome (Vaisvaser et al., 2016). Likewise, as a result of the complexity of miRNA–target interactions, miRNA can influence a person's response to stress. Accordingly, an individual's vulnerability to inherited disease and disorders may emerge because of an abnormal stress response. Consequently, the significance of genome information to human health and well-being should not be underrated (Hollins & Cairns, 2016).

In summary, this chapter on epigenetics enhances our knowledge of how individual health and therefore opportunity is influenced by early developmental events and earlier generations' environmental conditions. We learned that most epigenetic modulations may be altered, meaning that many can reasonably be reversed. Therefore, while adverse exposures can epigenetically program pathological stress-sensitivity through alterations in gene expression, it is believed that nurturing and safe environments will equally reestablish wellness and resilience. Importantly, the social determination of epigenetic traits commonly inherited shows that innate traits are not unavoidably impervious to social structures. Conley and Malaspina (2016) assert that this viewpoint relates to the earliest definition of health, identifying that people have the ability to adapt to changing environments. This information presents the moral obligation for health professionals to consider those mechanisms external to traditional settings (e.g., clinical) in which we encounter clients receiving services; specifically, structural limitations to their clients' health outcomes. Achieving optimal outcomes society-wide will necessitate an interdisciplinary and cross-sector approach. The current education of many health professionals to be culturally competent typically lacks recognition of the impact of social adversity on the impending risks for ailments and their outcomes for individuals they care for. Instead of the genetically deterministic structure that is frequently alluded to when educating students and endorsed indirectly by many practitioners, a socio-ecological model for the deviation from health comprises the consequences to exposure to environmental stressors. The optimal developmental trajectory across the life course happens on both a genetic and ideal environmental situation that dynamically channels a set of naturally programmed systems of maturation that lead to optimizing adult health. As an illustration, the developmental life course can be viewed as a ball plunging down a contoured surface, in which divergences from normal development can stem from environmental adversity, disease genes, or their interactions. These experiences can govern paths to pathology that are theoretically unalterable (Conley & Malaspina, 2016). The health professional's understanding that the environment can affect a person's health due to epigenetic processes should influence the professional's practices. Their actions should strive to promote the adaptive process (e.g., connecting people to proper authorities or community partners to improve their quality of life such as living conditions, educational advancement, etc.). Of note, addressing the social structures that disadvantage the health of individuals is crucial and includes both individualized treatments and advocacy for policy changes (Conley & Malaspina, 2016).

5

EARLY BRAIN DEVELOPMENT
Childhood trauma and adversity

The human brain is recognized as "the most complex three pounds in the universe" (Noble, 2014, p. 2). In fact, this classification does not seem outrageous given that we are born with 100 billion neurons at birth, and 250,000 to 500,000 new neurons are created every minute in the first couple months of an infant's life (Noble, 2014). Importantly, the human brain is structured in a hierarchical manner; however its development is influenced by genetics and experience (Bick & Nelson, 2016). Genetic developments prevail during most of the prenatal period; notably, environmental effects including exposure to maternal stress hormones, nutritive deficiencies, disease, or teratogens significantly sculpt prenatal brain development (Gaskill & Perry, 2014). In contrast, postnatal stages of brain development are profoundly influenced by experience. While genes afford a universal blueprint for brain development, with every person possessing a distinctive genetic plan, the environment governs the degree to which this blueprint is realized. Inherent here is that differences at the genomic level will affect how signals from the environment are used. Moreover, additional adaptations in the environment, and related feedback delivered to the brain, will influence patterns of gene expression that manage neural development (Gaskill & Perry, 2014). As noted by the National Academy of Sciences (2000), "Virtually every aspect of early human development, from the brain's evolving circuitry to the child's capacity for empathy, is affected by the environments and experiences that are encountered in a cumulative fashion, beginning early in the prenatal period and extending throughout the early childhood years" (p. 6). In this section, we will discuss elements pertaining to: (a) construction of the brain, (b) sensitive-critical periods of vulnerability, and (c) adversity as a barrier to brain development.

Construction of the brain

Human brain development is a complex process comprising the dynamic composition of gene expression. Development of the brain begins with the most fundamental systems including the brainstem and sensory motor areas and it concludes with the prefrontal cortex— the most complex region of the brain (Gaskill & Perry, 2014). The formation of the brain starts several weeks following conception, initially with creating the neural tube, followed by the production of varied brain cells including the neurons and glia (National Academy of Sciences, 2014). Once developed, these immature neurons initiate their travel to develop the cerebral cortex. The majority of cell migration accomplished prior to the mother completing her second trimester of pregnancy. Next, formation of the cerebral cortex occurs, which encompasses structured layers of neurons that are implicated in numerous facets of cognition, comprising information processing and memory storage. After immature neurons travel to their target destination, they differentiate by developing cell bodies and processes which are known as axons and dendrites (National Academy of Sciences, 2014).

When processes are formed, synapses, the connections between neurons that permit the communication of signals across the synaptic cleft, begin to form. In effect, these synapses are tiny areas that are between two brain cells that are next to each other, usually between a dendrite and an axon (National Academy of Sciences, 2014). Entire circuits are constructed, and after that neural networks are developed. Specifically, brain regions differ in the time point whereby peak synaptogenesis is attained (Bick & Nelson, 2016). Alteration of neuronal synapses occurs continually during one's lifetime. As research has established, more basic structures, for example, the visual cortex, reach peak synaptogenesis within the initial eight months of life (Bick & Nelson, 2016). The amount of synapses, or connections between neurons, becomes progressively complex in the first several years of life; specifically, a child has trillions of networks by age three (Noble, 2014). Conversely, more intricate structures in the prefrontal cortex attain their peak in about the 15th postpartum month (Bick & Nelson, 2016). As neurons are wired together in order to create a mature central nervous system circuit, a process of removing select synapses (i.e., synapse pruning) also takes place (Wu, Dissing-Olesen, MacVicar, & Stevens, 2015). The most robust growth and pruning of these connections take place in the initial three to four years of life, signifying that the brain is most plastic (i.e., capable of making new connections) in the early years of life (Noble, 2014). Given adults' highly dynamic neuronal circuitry systems, synaptic plasticity is customary with synaptic connections in numerous areas continuously going through remodeling based on experience (Wu et al., 2015). Consequently, reduced neuronal activity at synapses in both the emerging and adult nervous system has been associated with physical elimination of these less functional connections (Wu et al., 2015).

In the later stage of brain development, myelination occurs. Information transmitted along the length of the axon can occur quickly if they have a coating of myelin (fatty sheaf). In the final trimester of pregnancy, sensory and motor pathways start to myelinate, while association areas of the brain like the prefrontal cortex, continue to myelinate across the second decade of a person's life (National Academy of Sciences, 2014). Thus, the progression of myelination begins in the end of the second trimester, surges linearly across the first two decades of life, and ultimately carries on more slowly into middle adulthood (Bick & Nelson, 2016).

During brain development, it is important to acknowledge that the formation of neurons and their time-dependent connection into intricate functional circuits that traverse numerous neuronal layers need to be carefully regulated to support normal cortical function. Of relevance, white matter and grey matter are contained in the brain; axons or neural elements are the former and the majority of the rest of the brain is the latter.

Given the genetic-experiential (or intrinsic-extrinsic) influence and timing of production of synapses, we know that they are vastly overproduced early in a person's life course and mainly under genetic control; however pruning of synapses takes place largely after birth and is for the most part under experiential control (Bick & Nelson, 2016). Pruning enables brain networks to grow, fine-tune, and become more organized and efficient; thereby permitting the brain to mature in a manner that boosts its maximal acclimatization to the surrounding (Bick & Nelson, 2016). Accordingly, the prefrontal cortex of a child that is two-years of age is expected to have more synapses than the normal adult brain. However, during the course of the subsequent two to three decades, these synapses are pruned, returning to adult numbers, due mainly to experience; the prefrontal cortex reaches maturity at about 30 years of age. The plasticity and prolonged development of the brain provides an opportunity for continual modification of cognitive function, creating a potential vulnerability for the creation of abnormal circuitry producing compromised behavioral function (Kolb, Mychasiuk, & Gibb, 2014). The brain is especially vulnerable to experiences at the onset of puberty when the frontal lobe is massively pruning synapses (Kolb et al., 2014). For instance, being exposed to varied types of noise supports the development of neural circuitry, triggering auditory perception, which is essential for the advancement of higher order processes such as command of speech and language (Gaskill & Perry, 2014).

In summary, brain development is a lengthy process that extends beyond the mere unfolding of a genetic blueprint. Its development does not occur in a vacuum; rather it reveals a complex interaction of both genetic and experiential factors that influence the developing brain and eventually behavior. Brain development is depicted by intricate microstructural and macrostructural processes that include the emergence of the first neurons to the formation of the wholly operative adult brain—perhaps the most complex of biological systems. Revealing these intricate developments of the brain is central to understanding the creation of neural circuits and brain functions. Neurons are responsible for connections producing intricate, interconnected neural networks that underpin all human thought, feeling and action. As human beings we experience interactions that shape our brains throughout our lives. With maturation, brain regions are primed for higher cognitive functioning, which lasts for extended periods; therefore the phase for experience-dependent plasticity must be recognized.

The timing of environmental influence profoundly shapes the brain's potential for normative development; consequently sensitive and critical periods of development must be understood (Bick & Nelson, 2016). These periods are characteristically represented by a heightened degree of neuronal plasticity (i.e., the brain's ability to adapt and change), which advances the relevance of that opportunity (Cicchetti, Georgieff, Brunette, & Tran, 2015). Positive neuroplasticity is "the physiological ability of the brain to form and strengthen dendritic connections, produce beneficial morphological changes, and increase cognitive reserve" (Zmijewski, 2014, p. 1). Negative neuroplasticity is the "ability of the brain to atrophy and weaken dendritic connections, produce detrimental morphological changes, and decrease cognitive reserve" (Zmijewski, 2014, p. 1). Sensitive and critical periods happen early in life, traversing fetal and early postnatal periods. Incidents that take place during these periods affect brain function across the life span and possibly transgenerationally, which is recognized to precipitate developmental origins of adult health and disease (Cicchetti et al., 2015).

Sensitive periods, points in maturational growth when environmental information has a maximal effect on development, are perceived as a softer version of critical periods; that is, this is a period where the brain is mostly amenable to stimuli typically over a broad period of time (Cicchetti & Andersen, 2015). This heightened receptivity signifies an opportunity to create an improved (or worse) brain at stages where a person obtains more effect for specific stimuli than during other stages/time periods (Cicchetti et al., 2015). Sensitive periods indi-cate that there is a developmental phase of inherent competence for exchange between a human being and its environment. We know that experience-expectant learning (i.e., time when the brain is primed to certain aspects of environmental information) is most observed during sensitive periods. This is where a human being depends on particular kinds of experience in order to develop normally (Cicchetti et al., 2015). For example, nutrient and social stimulation affects function principally within the sensitive period time frame. Neural plasticity is also greater during a sensitive period than before or after the period; however, the system continues to be impressionable throughout development. Within the social domain a particularly compelling practice of an early sensitive period is imprinting, specifically filial or sexual imprinting (Baran, 2017). This imprinting is described as a form of learning that (a) can only occur during a limited period of time in a person's life, (b) is permanent, (c) comprises the learning of individual-specific characters, and (d) may happen when the proper behavior itself is not yet performed (Baran, 2017). Also, in general, among developing children the optimal window for environmental impact on hippocampal development is before the age of eight. Importantly, sensitive periods can be viewed as an enhanced opportunity for neural plasticity during development in contrast to critical periods, which are portrayed with greater determinism with regard to long-term neurobehavioral consequences (Cicchetti et al., 2015).

Critical periods are essential for the underpinning of constructing the human brain; this is a time with heightened neural plasticity during development. After critical periods cease, neural plasticity becomes quite low. Also, experience diminishes in its capacity to change neural circuits, although more contemporary research has ascertained mechanisms through which plasticity can be reestablished beyond the termination of a critical period (Hensch, 2016). This implies that abnormal neurodevelopmental results are not automatically irreversible (Hensch, 2016). Hartley and Lee (2015) assert that several developmental processes (sensory), including visual and auditory development and language attainment are dependent during the critical period. Specifically, the introduction of the critical period is driven by the initia-tion of sensory function, when peripheral sensory structures mature and start to transmit external sensory input into central structures. For instance, visual perception and ocular dominance in human beings is usually believed to close at approximately 7 years of age (Abuleil, 2017). The human brain's ability to restructure its connections in the visual cortex becomes progressively more problematic over the course of the person's life. Previously, developmental and neurological vision conditions (e.g., amblyopia), were considered endur-ing if they were not attended to during the critical period of brain development, attributable to the posited lack of plasticity in the adult brain (Abuleil, 2017). Importantly, while the opportunity of the critical period is fairly sudden, the closing is relatively slow and incom-plete, signifying that modifications can actually occur (Abuleil, 2017).

Through studying neurobiology of child development, it is important to learn how to acquire a measure of control as it relates to the timing of critical periods. This information can help to remedy overlooked opportunities or gaffes caused when connections are laid for a maturing nervous system. Hensch (2016) reported on a critical discovery that surfaced while inspecting an important signaling molecule in the brain. Specifically, GABA (gamma-ami-nobutyric acid), a neurotransmitter most recognized for compressing the firing of nerve cells, was found to play a crucial role in regulating when a critical period begins and ends. The parvalbumin-positive large basket cell, a GABA-producing neuron, most likely arranges the process (Hensch, 2016).

In summary, the process of early brain development is continually modified by stimuli within the environment. Experience is converted into blueprints of electrical activity within neural circuits; this electrical activity propels the various forms of plasticity that occur in a person's brain. Recognition of the dynamism of neural plasticity encompasses changes in the efficacy of already existing synaptic contacts, formation of new synaptic contacts or elimination of existing ones. These changes manifest both during development and later in life, although at a slower pace. Differences in the extent and enormity of plastic changes between the developing and the adult brain are related to sensitive and critical periods, preceded by age-specific elements and processes.

Adversity as a barrier to brain development

Early life adversities affect life course development, particularly when numerous adversities including poverty, nutritional deficiencies, high-crime communities, and low quality resources coincide (Black et al., 2017). For example, neuroscientific data has documented links between low socioeconomic status in early childhood and smaller hippocampal grey matter volume, which in unison with low frontal and temporal lobe volume, may well mediate links between poverty and low cognitive, academic, and behavioral performance (Black et al., 2017).

Andersen (2015) also reports that neuroanatomical research reveals that abuse that happens before puberty has more selective effects on the hippocampus, while abuse after puberty seems more selective for the prefrontal cortex in humans. Enhanced knowledge of the neurobiology of adversity (i.e., trauma) proposes convincing support of its long-term effect on the brain and body, as well as the considerable costs to society when trauma goes unaddressed. Recall that an event becomes traumatic when it inundates the neurophysiological system for coping with stress and causes the person to feel unsafe, vulnerable and unbridled (Clervil & DeCandia, 2013). What's more, traumatic experiences take place outside the sphere of customary experience; threaten one's physical, spiritual, and emotional well-being; and arouse intense feelings of powerlessness, fear, and lack of control (Clervil & DeCandia, 2013).

When confronted with a threat, structures in the limbic system (e.g., the amygdala and hypothalamus), which are the brain's emotional control center, trigger the body's survival responses. Specifically, the fight (aggressively tackling the basis of the stress), flight (evading the stress), and freeze (shutting down) responses can occur (De Bellis & Zisk, 2014). Additionally, neurohormones such as adrenaline and cortisol prime the body for battle to oppose the threat and defend itself. Later, these neurohormones can support the body's return to a functional state of balance when the threat has passed (Clervil & DeCandia, 2013). The stressors linked with a traumatic event are handled by the body's sensory systems via the brain's thalamus; in return this stimulates the amygdala, an essential part of the brain's fear detection and anxiety circuits. Moreover, cortisol levels are heightened through conduction of fear signals to neurons located in the hypothalamus, prefrontal cortex, and hippocampus; in addition, activity escalates in the locus coeruleus and sympathetic nervous system (De Bellis & Zisk, 2014). Following this, changes in catecholamine levels occur which promote changes in metabolic rate, heart rate, blood pressure, and alertness; subsequently, activation of other biological stress systems occurs (De Bellis & Zisk, 2014).

An individual can experience real and perceived threats which can continually retrigger the stress response, causing a person's neurological system to enter a state of disequilibrium. As a result of this persistently dysregulated state, a range of maladaptive behavioral responses can develop. Specifically, children subjected to early and continuous traumatic stress such as abuse, family violence, and neglect and lacking sufficient parental /adult supports are likely to experience toxic stress that has overwhelming effects on brain development (Clervil & DeCandia, 2013). It is evident that early life experiences have a huge impression on children's development. Specifically, developmental periods that occur between 0 and 5 years of age as well as those between 15 and 25 years of age are sensitive periods of human development with specific sections of the brain being more vulnerable to traumatic experiences. Black and colleagues (2017) also argue that children living in extreme poverty have an increased likelihood of exposure to multiple adversities (e.g., food insecurity, neglect, abuse, and exposure to violence) which tend to be intensified by living in communities with inadequate resources. These sustained experiences can modify brain construction and the functioning of neural pathways such as those related to learning, memory, and the capacity to self-regulate and cope. Furthermore, the person encountering this experience develops a heightened baseline state of physiological arousal as well as enhanced sensitivity to triggers (Clervil & DeCandia, 2013). These modifications position children at significant risk for unfavorable developmental, emotional, functional and academic outcomes. These experiences are also linked with difficulties with relations with friends, including undesirable externalizing behavior in school-age children and antisocial behavior and delinquency in adolescents that continues over time (Clervil & DeCandia, 2013). McEwen (2017) identifies that individuals who suffer extreme adversity experience an increased inflammatory response; this does not just occur in children but also in young adults contingent on their early life abuse. Furthermore, lifespan concerns regarding effects of being raised in poverty can extend to adulthood, having consequences with low task-related activation of brain areas supporting language, cognitive control and memory skills, and high activation of areas linked with emotional reactivity (Clervil & DeCandia, 2013).

A posited conduit in the link between childhood adversity and adult health is through modified hypothalamic-pituitary-adrenal axis feedback-loop functioning (Kuras et al., 2017). This is believed to occur as a result of biological programming, which takes place during sensitive periods in development, and regulates the function of stress systems. This programming arises very early in life, even prior to birth. For instance, exposure to smoking before birth (Stroud et al., 2014), environmental exposures, maternal stress and inadequate nutrition can change hypothalamic-pituitary-adrenal axis functioning in offspring (Kuras et al., 2017). Importantly, early childhood is a vital time for the development of the hippocampus. In fact, stress may affect the path of this development through glucocorticoid regulation of gene expression in the hippocampus. Adverse or traumatic environments can alter the functioning and size of the hippocampus, changing regulation of hypothalamic-pituitary-adrenal axis activity (Kuras et al., 2017). Glucocorticoid receptors are crucial regulators of hypothalamic-pituitary-adrenal feedback within the hippocampus; modifications in glucocorticoid receptors activity affects stress response. What's more, both prenatal and early childhood adversity are linked with variations in glucocorticoid receptors methylation and transcription. Thus, childhood adversity could bring about decreased hypothalamic-pituitary-adrenal axis feedback sensitivity, causing modified hypothalamic-pituitary-adrenal basal activity (Romens, McDonald, Svaren, & Pollak, 2015).

In summary, early human brain development constitutes a sequence of intricate processes resulting in the ontogeny of functionally operative neural circuits. Adverse exposures in early life, namely experiences such as child maltreatment, caregiver stress or depression and

6

DEVELOPMENTAL PSYCHOLOGY

Implications of ACEs

Developmental psychology is the study of change (growth and decline) as humans grow, mature, and gain experience with the world around them across the life course; though individuals may progress on broadly varying paths to arrive at comparable developmental endpoints (Paterson, Parish-Morris, Hirsh-Pasek, & Golinkoff, 2016). Change can appear rapidly or could surface progressively over time. There may also be a particular incipient event (e.g., trauma), or a collection of issues may interact to generate change (Paterson et al., 2016). Leeman (2018) recognizes that developmental psychology is deeply influenced by early and ongoing family relations and experiences that have a profound effect on later life displays of adjustment and functioning. Moreover, family experiences do not merely affect our own life course; we replicate our experiences in our offspring (i.e., intergenerational continuity). By using the lens of a developmental approach we will investigate the implications of ACEs on adult mental health considering the important interacting domains over time given that differences early in life (e.g., ACEs) can have cascading effects on later outcomes (e.g., adult mental health). ACEs heightens the likelihood for the development of stress and trauma-related psychological difficulties in adulthood. Specifically, Callaghan and Tottenham (2016) identify that early experiences establish the underpinning for life-long mental health; mental health is "a central determinant of individual well-being, family relationships, and engagement in society" (Rhodes, 2015, p. 1). As illustrated in this chapter, content will be reflective of Gillihan's (2018) message, "The more cogently we prove ourselves to have been shaped by causes, the more opportunities we create for changing" (p. ¶ 41).

Wounds inflicted on psychological health are important; however, their tendrils spread through an array of psychosocial and functioning spheres (Nurius, Green, Logan-Greene, & Borja, 2015). The effect of these underlying forces is frequently in progress before clinical symptoms are demonstrated. Efforts to understand the longer-term implications of ACEs bring forth the relevance of a life course lens that offers perspectives on cumulative adversity and how life pathways are primed and structured by various socially constructed developmental scaffolding and limitations (Halfon, Larson, Lu, Tullis, & Russ, 2014). Moreover, being perceptive and appreciating what developmental and behavioral health care professionals, especially pediatric practitioners, employ can be useful including: (a) recognizing major effects of the social environment and previous experiences on current behaviors; (b) appreciating the cumulative process on development and the enduring results of early disruptions; (c) acknowledging that maladaptive behaviors are frequently sustained because they were in fact adaptive at some time in the past; and (d) in general, thinking longitudinally over time (Nurius et al., 2015).

Importantly, ACEs in life not only carry developmental effects but also enhance risk of propagating a series of added stressors that can overpower individual coping and challenge recovery and health. By considering ACEs within a life course perspective (i.e., childhood, adolescent, and adulthood), it allows us to see how early childhood adversity conveys a distinctive ability to mar adult psychological well-being; this occurs both independent of and cumulative with other influential factors, such as social hardship and toxic stress as an adult (Nurius et al., 2015).

Childhood

Exposure to considerable childhood adversity impacts a daunting percentage of youth, comprising one of the most damaging effects on youth development. The prevalence of childhood adversity is high, approximately 50% in the US child population across numerous epidemiological surveys (McLaughlin, 2016). Research by Gilbert and colleagues (2015) as well as Ellis and Dietz (2017) reports that an estimated 60% of children reported at least one ACE; children of color are at highest risk. Interestingly, comparable prevalence assessments have been recorded in other high-income countries, in addition to in low- and middle-income countries worldwide (McLaughlin, 2016). ACEs comprise experiences including maltreatment, neglect, observed violence, and household dysfunctions, for example, parental mental ailments or substance abuse, and imprisonment of one or more family members; these indicate a range of conditions depicted by multiple forms of chronic and acute stress.

More specifically, Valentino (2017) reported that an estimated 3.9 million children were subjects of abuse accounts to child welfare organizations and approximately 700,000 cases were validated, contributing to a countrywide victimization rate of 9 per 1,000 children (US Department of Health and Human Services (US DHHS), 2015; Valentino, 2017). Significantly, over 90% of abused children are injured by one or both parents (US DHHS, 2015; Valentino, 2017). Consequently, child abuse can be described as a pathogenic relational experience often taking place in the parent-child relationship. Thus, considering child abuse and neglect, the maladaptive character of the parent-child relationship is fundamentally able to heighten risk for psychopathology as well as other undesirable abnormalities for maltreated children (Valentino, 2017).

Formative early childhood periods of psychological development can be challenging and have a debilitating impact on a child's emotional health, especially when approaches to coping or defense are limited and exposure to ACEs is amplified by lack of social support (Beutel et al., 2017). Social supports are critical to psychological development, given that they modify the risk associated with childhood trauma. Social support and the interaction of individual behavioral styles (child temperament) also influence the severity of the long-term mental health consequences. For example, a young child with a hereditary propensity to fearfulness has a heightened chance to develop anxiety or depression than a child lacking that susceptibility. This is remarkably powerful in the context of cruel, unreliable relationships and experiences, including those linked with poor quality child care by the family/guardian, or a depressed mother or father. That said, early adversity represents a *signature* that liberates a child's hereditary predisposition for anxiety, constructing a brain that reacts to lower intensities of stress with extreme fear and anxiety, creating lifelong effects for mental health (National Scientific Council on the Developing Child, 2012).

Likewise, another example of social support and ACEs relates to attachment. Immature human beings such as young children are more vulnerable for extended periods of their lives than any other species. This dependency has required an all-embracing attachment system between adults and children that causes overwhelming deficiencies whenever the young child does not receive this type of protection (Bloom, 2013). Exposure to early child separation due to parental incarceration and child trauma is embedded in attachment theory (Arditti, 2012). Attachment, an essential emotional bond between child and caregiver (e.g., parent/guardian), operates as a foundation for future relationships and development. Healthy attachment relationships experienced by children are deemed to function as a basis for self-organization and physiological self-regulation and to encourage development of self-control and social skills (Arditti, 2012; Bowlby, 1982). Bonds like this could be regarded as a safe refuge for children; healthy bonds foster self-assurance and the capability to explore and gain meaningful understanding of the world, along with safety during periods of anguish. ACEs that reduce or eradicate the availability of an attachment figure are crucial since these ACEs may well intensify a child's susceptibility to subsequent adversity (Arditti, 2012). Attachment troubles can increase the likelihood that the child will encounter comparable experiences throughout their life on the basis of actions that surface from former attachment disruptions (Arditti, 2012; Bowlby, 1982). Parental incarceration can potentially be linked with disturbances in attachment bonds, given the physical separation caused by the parent's imprisonment along with disjointedness in the child's care—especially if the imprisoned parent was a main caregiver preceding his or her incarceration (Arditti, 2012). This reality presents a specific setback for modern family configurations merely because previously there was a higher caregiver to child quotient than occurs today (Bloom, 2013). Due to the nature of our world, children have fewer occasions to bond with dependable, consistent, and available adults (Bloom, 2013). Attachment theory hypothesizes that real-life experiences that disturb attachment bonds or pose a possibility of disruption cause acute anxiety for children and grief after removal of the parent/guardian (Bowlby, 1982).

As it relates to cumulative ACEs, it is important to recognize that varied childhood adversities tend to co-occur. Thus, moving attention to include not just singular but cumulative forms of exposure is requisite. Exposure to these adversities produces step-dose patterns in which greater exposure to numerous forms of stressful experiences is linked with a broader range of impaired mental health, to accumulated stress burden, and to experiences of social and behavioral difficulties throughout youth and into adulthood (McLaughlin, 2016; Nurius et al., 2015). Given this information, it is easy to see why early life adversities operate as primary stressors that establish the platform for and interact with secondary stressors in the form of additional adversities. Consequently, these developments flow through various life domains across the life course including education, work, and relationship thus connecting chains of risk and producing interconnected adversities that link ACEs and later life outcomes (Nurius et al., 2015). Even more broadly, ACEs or more general child trauma (e.g., accidents, witnessing accidents, natural disasters, refugee status, sexual victimization, terrorism, and acts of war) contributed to over 6.5 million referrals to child protection agencies for abuse and neglect in the United States in 2013, according to the most recent report of the U.

S. Department of Health and Human Services (US DHHS, 2015). In the United Kingdom, trauma led to the referral of 390,000 children to care services in 2014–2015, according to the National Society for the Prevention of Cruelty to Children (NSPCC, 2016). The NSPCC estimates that for every child identified as abused and neglected, eight remain unidentified. More than 70% of these children have experienced two or more traumatic life events (Lyons-Ruth & Jacobvitz, 2008), and up to 90% of them have disorganized styles of attachment (Gilgun & Hirschey, 2017).

Young children respond to trauma events differently than adults since their brains are not fully developed. For example, a toddler who is coping with ACEs behaves differently compared to an adolescent who has experienced numerous ACEs because of dissimilar psychological abilities, emotional requirements, and social experiences at diverse ages. Similarly, young children display symptoms of depression or post-traumatic stress disorder (PTSD) differently as compared to young adults (National Scientific Council on the Developing Child, 2012). Salloum and colleagues (2018) argue exposure to multiple ACEs in young children is linked with increased risk of PTSD, post-traumatic stress severity, and more internalizing and externalizing behavioral problems compared to young children with no ACEs exposure. Leeman (2018) also reports that children afflicted by ACEs experience higher levels of major depression, attention deficit hyperactivity disorder, PTSD, conduct disorder and oppositional defiant disorder compared to children who have not experienced ACEs. Dudley (2015) further notes that children exposed to ACEs become hypervigilant; they are continuously anticipating something bad to occur to them and they frequently perceive danger where none exists. These young children not only have a tendency to be hyperreactive to perceived threats of danger, they also strive not to reflect on their traumatic experiences and they become distraught when those experiences occur (Dudley, 2015). Moreover, other experiences that prompt them to recall previous traumatic experiences, or epitomize those experiences, intensify these and other trauma-related symptoms that have developed (Dudley, 2015). Of note, young children likewise have trouble relaxing themselves once hyperreactivity has been activated (Dudley, 2015). While these complications may perhaps be obvious to others who know them, these affected children are much too young to understand that they are experiencing psychiatric problems. What's more, when ACEs are chronic and severe, a child may experience dissociation (Leeman, 2018). This can occur at the time of overpowering experiences of abuse and neglect; ironically dissociation can serve to protect the child from a fragmentation of the self via numerous disconnections in the self. This happens at both mental and bodily levels (Leeman, 2018). Coincidentally, dissociation can be regarded as an adaptive coping strategy in conditions of severe trauma, yet problematic when used for extended periods.

Hodges and colleagues (2013) discovered that for children 8–12 years of age, the quantity of varied interpersonal traumatic events was significantly correlated with trauma-related symptoms including posttraumatic stress, anxiety, depression, dissociation, anger, and sexual concerns. Interestingly, research reports that the type of ACE a child experiences may well bring about different trauma-related complications. For instance, Briggs-Gowan and colleagues (2010) found that exposure to interpersonal violence among young children aged two and three years was linked with disruptive behaviour, depression, and anxiety, whereas involvement in non-interpersonal violence was linked with anxiety. All of these behaviors can adversely impact learning and progression in school.

In summary, young children who are exposed to ACEs are vulnerable to experiencing unfavorable psychological sequela (e.g., emotional and behavioral challenges) and struggle in school as they go through a relatively quick developmental period, have inadequate coping skills, and are strongly reliant on their primary caregiver (e.g., parent) to safeguard their well-being. Factors that heighten poor psychological development are important to recognize, including limited supportive relationships with one or more adults, having insecure attachment relationships, and a child's limited early life intrapersonal skills. Repeated or continuous activation from exposure to ACEs can interrupt not only customary physical but also psychological development and can furthermore alter the brain's architecture. Healthy social support and relationships from adults are among the most important actions to reduce both the biological effects of stress overload and to promote positive cognitive and emotional processing (Nurius et al., 2015). Other resilience factors, preventive and early intervention strategies will be discussed in later chapters.

BOX 6.1 CASE ILLUSTRATION: 5-YEAR-OLD

Background

- 5-year-old female presents for a visit with a complaint of pain in right ear
- This is her first visit to see you
- She recently moved to this town after her parents got divorced

Past medical history

- 28-year-old mother with good prenatal care
- 39 weeks' gestational age
- Uncomplicated birth
- Immunizations are up-to-date

Family history

- Mother recently started working full-time after divorce from husband
- Mother reports there was domestic violence in the marriage
- Child often spends time at her maternal grandparents' house when the mother works late
- Child's father lives two hours away and she only sees him every other weekend

Social history

- Mother grew up living with a father who is an alcoholic and he still drinks
- Mother was diagnosed with Attention Deficit Hyperactivity Disorder when 10 years old
- Child's father grew up in a home with domestic violence
- Mother's job is stressful and she has trouble sleeping; reports feeling worried and depressed

- Child misses her former daycare center and is "acting out" in her present day care; often complains of stomach aches and wanting to go home

Physical exam

- Weight: 40 pounds (>95 percentile). Height: 39 inches (>75 percentile). Basal Metabolic Index: 18.5
- General: displays anxious behaviors; clings to mother; sucks thumb at times
- Head, eyes, ears, neck, throat: normal; pupils equal, round, reactive to light and accommodation; moist mucous membranes; left tympanic membrane scarred, right ear is red with pus
- Chest: expiratory wheezing; normal breathing; no rales
- Cardiac: normal S1 and S2; normal rate and rhythm; no murmur audible
- Abdomen: bowel sounds, non-tender, non-distended
- Skin: rough, red, dry patches on left arm

Discussion questions

- What other information would you like to have and why?
- What risks to child's health have you identified and why are they risks?
- What is the child's Adverse Childhood Experiences score at time of the visit per mother's account of family history? What are the co-occurring adversities you can identify?
- What opportunities to promote wellness and healthy development have already been missed?
- Can you identify behaviors that may be responses to stress and adversity?
- How might you discuss stress, adverse experiences and risk as well as resilient factors with this child's mother?
- What are your recommendations moving forward? For child? For mother?

Adolescents

Adolescence is a critical developmental phase that functions as a passage to adulthood. Recognizing risks such as exposure to ACEs for challenging adolescent transitions to adulthood is of significant importance since trajectories formed at some stages are deeply related to well-being in later adulthood. The prevalence of ACEs is higher in adolescents than in younger children; however it is not as likely to be reported (Flaherty et al., 2013). For example, the Fourth National Incidence Survey of Child Abuse and Neglect discovered that an estimated 21 out of 1000 adolescents 12 to 14 years of age were abused compared to 8.5 out of 100 children zero to two years of age (Flaherty et al., 2013). Notably, roughly eight out of 1000 of these adolescent cases were in fact turned into the child protective services for maltreatment. Under-reporting might be attributable to suppositions that ACEs are less damaging for adolescents compared to younger children (Flaherty et al., 2013). Soleimanpour, Geierstanger, and Brindis (2017) found that over half (54%) of all adolescents 12 to

17 years of age in the United States have been subjected to at least one ACE, and an esti-mated one-quarter (28%) experienced two or more ACEs.

Specific subgroups of adolescents confront increased risks, such as youth who are lesbian, gay, bisexual, transgender, or questioning as well as adolescents who are imprisoned or involved in the juvenile justice system (Soleimanpour et al., 2017). Adolescent ACEs have been associated with adverse psychological and behavioral health concerns such as depressed mood, anxiety, Post-Traumatic Stress Disorder symptoms, risk-taking behavior, eating dis-orders, substance use, and suicide attempts (Flaherty et al., 2013).

Normally, in early adolescence or middle grades years, there is enormous growth physically, socially, intellectually, emotionally and spiritually. Puberty and a host of psychosocial changes linked with developing an increasingly cultivated identity, unearthing personal abilities, inter-ests, and skills are essential during this time period. Moreover, establishing meaningful peer and intimate relationships, bearing responsibility for more autonomous and adult decisions regarding risks, health, and the future are prime during adolescence. This exhilarating stage of develop-ment is exemplified by discovery and rapidly increasing capacities but it is likewise associated with many factors that render adolescents to be highly vulnerable (Mann, Kristjansson, Sigfus-dottir, & Smith, 2014). Also, conscious personal awareness and self-conscious peer comparison can add to the stressfulness of this life stage (Mann et al., 2014).

Socio-emotional portions of the brain dominate thinking and are related to emotional, frequently intense, reactions to stressful life experiences such as ACEs. This is reflected in life course development as individuals age from middle school to become high school and col-lege students; the prefrontal cortex develops and the cognitive control functions of the brain assume greater influence, which impacts psychological outcomes during extreme adverse experiences. Importantly, these cognitive control functions are linked with an increasing capability for logic (i.e., evaluating the pros and cons of a certain response) and formulating precise plans concerning the future. Additionally, as the prefrontal cortex matures, an ado-lescent's capacity also develops to disregard early fight or flight responses, permitting more mature reactions to difficult life experiences (Mann et al., 2014).

Once an individual reaches adolescence, they are at risk of experiencing at least one trau-matic event (Macdonald, Danielson, Resnick, Saunders, & Kilpatrick, 2010), and when contrasted to adulthood, trauma exposure is at its apex at this stage. This highpoint of exposure is presented in research, with higher rates of PTSD discovered in adolescents (13%), contrasted to adults (7 %) (Breslau, Wilcox, Storr, Lucia, & Anthony, 2004). Millions of adolescents who have been exposed to ACEs (e.g., substance abuse among adults in the home, maltreatment, and community violence) are susceptible to taking part in higher rates of substance use, aggression, and other aberrant behavior compared with their unexposed and less-exposed peers (Brumley, Jaffee, & Brumley, 2017). Adolescents subjected to ACEs demonstrate high levels of hopelessness and cynical beliefs about their future academic attainment, such as being able to gain advanced schooling (Brumley et al., 2017). Solei-manpour and colleagues (2017) also found that ACE afflicted adolescents have a greater chance of repeating an academic level in school, having reduced resilience, heightened pos-sibility for learning and behavioral problems, suicidal ideation, and early initiation of sexual pursuits and pregnancy. Actually, there is a greater prevalence of these undesirable effects among adolescents 12 to 17 years of age after experiencing more than one ACE (Solei-manpour et al., 2017). Of those adolescents with ACE counts of three or more, close to half (48%) of adolescents experience low engagement in school, 44% do not have an ability to remain calm and controlled, and 41% display high externalizing behaviors (Soleimanpour et al., 2017). Moreover, there is an increased risk of adolescents with a history of ACEs meeting the diagnostic criteria for not only individual disorders but also comorbidity across disorder categories (Mcchesney, Adamson, & Shevlin, 2015).

Adolescents whose childhood ACEs have gone unchecked may well experience developmental symptoms including uncertainty in their sense of self (Dudley, 2015). Lacking parental nurture and support, this unstable sense of self can be so excessive that on occasion the adolescent feels desolate. This emptiness can be accompanied by cutting, in order to sense pain and see the bleeding; likewise, comparable behavior can surface in an effort to feel something and discern that they are alive (Dudley, 2015). Relational problems are also common and characterized by intense but volatile relationships. These relational struggles are due, to a certain extent, to a desperate need for attachments to feel whole, in consort with fears of abandonment. These complexities are also caused by rapidly alternating discernments of significant others, which alter from idealizing them to debasing them, due to feelings that the other individual does not care about them (Dudley, 2015). Interestingly, the nature of our societies encourages adolescents to have considerably fewer opportunities to bond with dependable, trustworthy, and available adults (Bloom, 2015). This failing grows to be a more pervasive dilemma in adolescence when the yearning to become more independent from primary caregivers is developmentally normal but the only available relational alternates are peers (Bloom, 2013). ACE afflicted adolescents also experience problems in normalizing their mood due to extreme depressive, irritable, or anxious responses to non-traumatic circumstances. This mood volatility can give rise to suicidal behavior, misplaced and forceful surges of anger, or trouble in managing anger. Furthermore, ACE-afflicted adolescents may display impulsive, possibly self-damaging behavior (e.g., uncontrolled sex and substance abuse); when under extreme stress, these adolescents can for a short time become paranoid or experience dissociative symptoms (e.g., not sensing control of one's body or actions) (Dudley, 2015). Broad-based instabilities like these bring about substantial emotional anguish and dysfunction. It is not uncommon for ACE-afflicted adolescents in these situations to try to suppress or disguise this penetrating anxiety and fear with a hard, *it doesn't matter to me,* veneer. When this cover is linked with the problem in handling anger and impulsivity that are part of this collection of developmental adversities, these adolescents can seem hostile and intimidating (Dudley, 2015).

Lastly, Andrews and colleagues' research (Andrews, Jobe-Shields, López, & Metzger, 2015) indicates that disparities in ACE exposure chiefly accounts for racial and ethnic disparities in trauma-related psychological status. Adolescents from low-income families with a history of ACEs show greater risk of deleterious mental health outcomes compared to adolescents from high-income families. Comparably, Balistreri and Alvira-Hammond's (2016) research reported that non-Hispanic Black adolescents are more likely to experience any ACE (68.8%) when contrasted to non-Hispanic other (57.8%), non-Hispanic white (52.4%) or Hispanic adolescents (58.2%). Importantly, they also recognized that family functioning (i.e., positive parent-child relations) lessened the adverse impact of cumulative ACEs on adolescent health and emotional well-being (Balistreri & Alvira-Hammond, 2016). Positive family functioning operates as a way of protection when confronted with hardship and diminishes the harmful relationship between other adverse characteristics (e.g., parental divorce and adolescent mental health) (Balistreri & Alvira-Hammond, 2016). Similarly, López and colleagues (2017) report that evaluations of ACE exposure indicate that non-Hispanic Black and Hispanic adolescents experience greater interpersonal violence (e.g., physical abuse) compared to non-Hispanic white youth. Along with experiencing more traumatic events, contrasted to non-Hispanic Whites, racial and ethnic minority adolescents endure greater resource-related problems that surface to exacerbate post-traumatic responding. Specifically, these adolescents deal with more post-trauma loss, less access to trauma-related psychological services, and extended periods of enduring symptoms if untreated. Thus, adolescents with limited resources may have encumbered recovery from ACEs and consequently increase their chance of acquiring later mental health struggles (Andrews et al., 2015).

In summary, adolescent exposure to ACEs is quite common; what's more, ACEs are irrefutably a developmental risk and, consequently, are fundamental to mental health for adolescents. Over 50% of adolescents have reportedly been subjected to ACEs. This exposure can have damaging consequences, such as heightened probability for learning and behavioral concerns and suicidal ideation. Adolescence is a distinctive developmental phase of fast growth during which physiologic, intellectual, social, and emotional adaptations appear simultaneously. Adolescents subjected to ACEs are less capable of effectively traversing this transformational phase on account of detrimental outcomes of traumatic experiences on their emotional and cognitive development and/or lack of or inadequate positive supports.

Adulthood

ACEs are ever-present exposures that interact with life course events that heighten the chance of acute psychopathology and alter mental health trajectories of adults (Fink & Galea, 2015). In Kessler and colleagues (2010), the World Health Organization assesses that 30% of adult mental illness in 21 countries may well be credited to ACEs. Psychological development and changes that occur evolve through a lifelong process with experiences from childhood likely affecting psychological well-being throughout adult years—midlife and beyond (Infurna, Rivers, Reich, & Zautra, 2015). ACEs not only have detrimental effects during childhood and adolescence, these adversities can leave a scar into midlife and old age (Infurna et al., 2015). ACEs are linked with less emotional support and more stress in social relationships in adult life, lower levels of well-being, and premature onset of functional limitations, ailments, and early death (Infurna et al., 2015). Moreover, irrespective of the ACEs an adult experienced, data infers that an increasing number of adverse experiences during childhood relate not only to deterioration of physical health but also mental health outcomes in adulthood (Iniguez & Stankowski, 2016). Furthermore, the increasing number of adverse experiences an adult is afflicted with during childhood promotes an intergenerational cycle of ACE-related mental health, behavioral and social problems (Iniguez & Stankowski, 2016).

In adults, a history of ACEs has been associated with numerous disorders including mood, personality, anxiety, substance abuse, and impulse control (Green et al., 2010; Leeman, 2018; Putnam, Harris, & Putnam, 2013). The original ACE study speaks to a dose-response relationship. Varied substance use behaviors have been recognized as ACE consequences, such as prematurely starting alcohol use (Dube et al., 2006), problematic drinking behavior into adulthood (Dube, Anda, Felitti, Edwards, & Croft, 2002), intense smoking during adulthood (Ford, Zhao, Tsai, & Li, 2011), prescription drug use (Anda, Brown, Felitti, Dube, & Giles, 2008), and illegal drug use self-reported addiction (Dube et al., 2003). Fink and Galea (2015) allege that many ACEs are correlated exposures that can start a chain of risk all through life. For instance, while child abuse directly heightens risk of psychopathology in the injured party, those who suffer from ACEs are considerably more likely to experience adulthood trauma, signifying this cycle of trauma may well start early and be perpetuated during the life course. In addition, there is strong substantiation that persons afflicted by interpersonal traumas at any age have a two-to-three-fold greater risk of experiencing a second trauma; nearly one in four college rape victims report multiple instances of victimization in the past year, though 45% of all rapes conveyed in this research sample happened among the 3% of women who recounted three or more sexual victimizations (Fink & Galea, 2015).

Psychiatric illnesses, particularly depression and PTSD in adulthood, have been found to be associated with higher ACE scores (Chapman et al., 2004; Widom, DuMont, & Czaja, 2007). While PTSD is acknowledged in the Diagnostic and Statistical Manual of Mental Disorders, 5th edition as a possible result of uncompromising single-event traumas (American Psychiatric Association, 2013), not all early life trauma is correspondingly linked with PTSD in adulthood (Leeman, 2018; Pratchett & Yehuda, 2011). Compared to adults with a past of single-event trauma during childhood, PTSD is more widespread in adults with a past of ACEs (Leeman, 2018; Pratchett & Yehuda, 2011). Pratchett and Yehuda (2011) advise that revictimization, along with other personal characteristics, elucidates variance in outcomes in the development of PTSD following ACEs. Importantly, attachment predicts severity of PTSD symptoms among adults afflicted with ACEs.

To first gain insights on adult attachment, Ogle and colleagues report (Ogle, Rubin, & Siegler, 2015) that adult attachment style denotes systematic patterns of expectations, viewpoints, and emotions regarding the accessibility and receptiveness of those near to us during times of hardship. Bowlby (1982) conveys that attachment patterns are developed during early experiences with caregivers and preserved by future interpersonal relations in adulthood. In due time, these beliefs become adopted and form mental depictions of the self and others in intimate relationships. Consequently, this informs how people sense and cope with real and perceived dangers throughout the life course (Ogle et al., 2015). Disruptions to early attachment relationships associated with experiences of ACEs may worsen the effect of experiences of chronic or cumulative ACEs or subsequent victimization (Pratchett & Yehuda, 2011). Attachment research indicates that parents' recollections of their personal early attachment experiences affect their parenting attachment behavior with their child (Pratchett & Yehuda, 2011). Second-generation effect is the term used by Hesse and Main (2006) to describe how children of abused parents exhibited disorganized attachment behavior. Interestingly, disorganized child attachment was not perceived as a reaction to direct abuse experiences; however, instead it was related to the parental traumatic experience being unintegrated. Parents were frightful as a result of their unresolved trauma. In this fright, the parents conduct themselves in either frightened or frightening ways (Hesse & Main, 2006). When looking at older adults and attachment, Ogle and colleagues (2015) report that insecure attachment (i.e., anxiety and avoidance combined) is a strong predictor of PTSD symptoms in those afflicted with a wide-range of ACEs. Furthermore, Ogle et al.'s (2015) research displayed that the proportion of variance in PTSD symptoms described by insecure attachment doubled among older adults with existing PTSD symptoms due to ACEs compared to older adults who conveyed symptoms associated with traumas that surfaced in adulthood. This outcome was directed by an increase in the predictive utility of attachment anxiety among older adults with early life traumas. Contrasted to adulthood traumas, ACEs may be more prone to interrupt the development of secure attachment, which may hinder the development of effective approaches for controlling negative affect and coping with stress, thus intensifying older adults' vulnerability to PTSD.

From a developmental psychological perspective, ACEs undermine learning and academic achievement, compromising achievement in adulthood across academic, workforce, and socioeconomic spheres (Nurius et al., 2015). Consequently, this undermined success produces contexts partial toward exposure to further social stressors, a scarcity of social and personal resources, as well as adult mental disorders (Nurius et al., 2015). Increased exposure to later undesirable life events may show up in many forms, for example, relationship difficulties, housing insecurity, disability and contact with the criminal justice system (Nurius et al., 2015).

Notably, Kim, Park, and Kim (2016) state that one harmful outcome of ACEs is that those wounded are prone to display a number of socio-behavioral challenges, and consequently become perpetrators of misconduct. Specifically, being afflicted with ACEs considerably heightens the risk of misconduct in adulthood. From a developmental perspective, many changes occur in early life (even prenatally) that inform adulthood; specifically, serotonergic function is vital for the management of emotional responses, impulsivity, and aggression. Conceivably, this epigenetic change leads to the continuation of poor mental health effects and social regulation in adults (DeLisi & Vaughn, 2015; De Sanctis, Nomura, Newcorn, & Halperin, 2012). Smith, Park, Ireland, Elwyn, and Thornberry (2013) reported that ACE-afflicted children are two to six times more liable to develop criminal behavior in young adulthood, compared to those with no exposure to ACEs. For instance, Stouthamer-Loeber, Loeber, Homish, and Wei (2001) examined the relationship between ACEs and criminal behavior over three developmental periods (i.e., adolescence, early adulthood, adulthood) in the National Youth Survey, and discovered that ACEs were substantially related to involvement in criminal behavior that remained into adulthood across crime types, counting index crimes and intimate partner violence.

Lastly, we know that ACEs disrupts the construction of social bonds and is linked with reduced familial social support (Lee et al., 2017). These disruptions create vulnerabilities to homelessness throughout the life course by limiting educational and employment options, increasing risk for criminal justice system involvement and later life victimization, and decreasing the probability of forming marital bonds. These may contribute to homelessness directly by forming impediments to employment and housing or indirectly by reducing the ability for the person to survive income devastations, inexpensive housing, or manage health crises via familial support (Lee et al., 2017). Moreover, ACEs have been related to poorer psychiatric outcomes among a sample of homeless women under age 50 and among homeless adults with mental ailments. Older homeless adults who were afflicted by ACEs have a correspondingly high prevalence of ACEs, as do younger homeless populations (Lee et al., 2017; Tam, Zlotnick, & Robertson, 2003). Specifically, these authors found a dose-response relationship between ACEs and psychiatric morbidities, in spite of the high prevalence of both ACEs and psychiatric illnesses. According to the Morbidity and Mortality Weekly Report (Centers for Disease Control and Prevention (CDC), 2010), the prevalence of childhood physical abuse was higher in these homeless adults than in the general population (33.3% versus 14.8%); yet Lee and colleagues (2017) found that it was similar to a national sample of younger homeless adults. Slopen et al. (2016) also discovered a high prevalence of parental death occurring during homeless adults' childhood when compared to the general population (21.4% versus 0.3%). Premature parental demise may have ramifications on later development, in view of the psychological and economic effect on the family system. Edalati and colleagues (2017) further account that having a history of a specific ACE (childhood physical abuse) in homeless adults has been found to significantly heighten the risk of aberrant behaviors, arrest, imprisonment, and damaging police encounters among homeless individuals; this is evident even after controlling for the significant effect of drug use and abnormal survival behaviors. What's more, other ACEs have been implicated with increasing the risk of criminal justice involvement among adults who suffer homelessness. Thus, early exposure to ACEs likely has a long-term effect on individuals' proclivity to become involved in the criminal justice system later in life.

Unsurprisingly, the adverse effects of life stress among the homeless can result from exposure to many forms of ACEs. These stressful events can be viewed as chains of risk whereby one exposure often produces another in probabilistic instead of deterministic ways (Padgett, Smith, Henwood, & Tiderington, 2012). While taking a life course perspective, it is important to remember that there are numerous points for health prevention and intervention. Thinking systematically, it's crucial to consider beyond individual-level factors but to also recognize upstream factors that produce and sustain inequalities, intensifying the accrual of adversities among those that have reduced resources and resilience capacity (Nurius et al., 2015).

In summary, ACEs have their roots in the initial years of life; however, they have significant effects on developmental aspects of an adult's psychological process. Attachment is a vital aspect of human development having profound influence on adult psychological responses to toxic stress and adversity as well as intergenerational implications. PTSD, homelessness, and criminal justice concerns are but a few areas that heighten poorer psychological outcomes. These are some population groups that are subjected to enduring adversity. Next we will broaden this lens by examining implications of ACEs from a community and structural perspective; this perspective on ACEs and inequalities forthwith holds that differences in the socioeconomic conditions, at all stages of the life-course, cause differences in a myriad of health outcomes. Also, while the number and severity of ACEs makes a person's survival extraordinary in itself, in later chapters we will discuss the relevance of resilience and change that occurs through human strength.

7

COMMUNITY AND STRUCTURAL DETERMINANTS

Implications of ACEs

People are often acquainted with the African proverb "it takes a village to raise a child," which emphasizes the vital role that the entire community takes in promoting the well-being of children. It is a logical conclusion then that, "If it takes a village to raise a child, it takes a village to abuse a child" (Word Press, 2017, ¶1). Brandon Jones (2013) furthers this premise by concluding, "The village that hides the truth cannot expect to heal, but to pass on the pain" (¶20). Thus, the question arises, "*what support and infrastructure do communities require in order to fulfill this role*" (Raising the Village, 2013, p. 7)? It is within this community context that the safety and welfare of children and families must be understood (Raising the Village, 2013). Consequently, looking closely at community determinants (i.e., social, economic and environmental circumstances that shape child and family well-being) is important (Raising the Village, 2013). These are structural factors that tend to be beyond the control of individuals; specifically, the community or population features are of critical importance, not merely individual or family characteristics. Accordingly, ACEs persist not just because of individual or family conditions (downstream) however but also due to upstream factors— macro level factors including government policies, social, physical, economic and environmental factors that affect health. Upstream factors produce and maintain inequities, intensifying the accumulation of ACEs among those that have lesser resources and resilience capacity (Nurius et al., 2015). While these upstream factors have demonstrable power, they are often perceived in less direct ways yet significantly influence a person's opportunities across the life course.

As noted by Bruner (2017), the influential ACEs research initiated in a medical context was individual focused. The original research indicators used were formed and mainly employed to measure ACEs that did not take into account community or structural determinants of health. Specifically, these indicators relate to the immediate family home environment and to particular events of disruption to the safety within that home setting (Bruner, 2017). Consequently, ACEs research outcomes directed attention to look at affording access to medical care and more recently to (a) extend attention to address health disparities and (b) expand attention to children's healthy development and the social determinants of health to optimize population health (Bruner, 2017). Above all, findings from ACEs research appeals for a far broader emphasis on the effects of the family, community, and social determinants of health on healthy child development across the life course (Bruner, 2017). Importantly, even when families can provide a safe haven in their homes, children can be subjected to adversity outside the household that influences their healthy development (Bruner, 2017; Lewis, 2009). It is essential to understand the community and structural level determinants and how power relations relate to impinge on lived experiences of individuals affected by ACEs and the capacity to achieve positive social change (Pyle, Golderer, & Hargro, 2016).

Community

Halfon and colleagues (Halfon, Larson, Son, Lu, & Bethell, 2017) argue that the role of community context is no more powerfully represented than in the social determinants of health—i.e., "the conditions in which people are born, grow, live, work and age (Braveman & Gottlieb, 2014, p. 19)." Similarly, Healthy People 2020 describe the social determinants of health as factors that shape one's access to the best health and longevity including neighborhood and built environment, economic stability, health and health care, education, and social and community context (Office of Disease Prevention and Health Promotion, 2018). Genetic vulnerabilities interact with these environmental variables (e.g., toxic stress, toxins, crowding, noise, destitute living conditions, unfit and low quality schools, and unsafe workplaces) to create either wellbeing or ill health. People are born into and mature in these spaces across the life course (Halfon et al., 2017). Given the relevance of ACEs and their involvement in the progress of risk factors for poor health, exposure to ACEs should be acknowledged as a social determinant of health (Monnat & Chandler, 2014).

ACEs linked with community and societal actions influence individuals at all social strata, however, individuals with low economic resources often have higher ACEs (Tomer, 2014). Halfon, Larson, Son, Lu, and Bethell (2017) reported that contemporary work by the World Health Organization Commission on Social Determinants of Health in addition to the Robert Wood Johnson Foundation Commission to Build a Healthier America have underscored how the allocation of health disparities and income inequality are inextricably linked. They also note how central this underlying link can be early in the life course. Halfon et al.'s (2017) research showed how risks for ACEs take place at each stratum of the income hierarchy and not merely affecting those below the level of poverty. In line with the income modeling of other health risks, progressing up the gradient reveals that individuals further up the income bracket enjoy greater levels of health and reduced levels of adversity (Halfon et al., 2017). For families who are financially impoverished, limited economic resources, and inadequate support for child development produce little time and income available for relevant endeavors such as quality childcare, kindergarten, and enriching, rousing activity which pushes their children to join schools with low human capital (Tomer, 2014). Moreover, families who experience such circumstances have an elevated rate of family separation or divorce and dysfunction producing high rates of ACEs (Tomer, 2014).

Communities, especially communities of color and low-income communities, accumulate an overwhelming number of risk factors for ACEs (Cohen, Davis, & Realini, 2016). The United States poorest census tracts unduly include people of color. Accordingly, 81.3% of children living in census tracts with poverty rates greater than 50% are children of color; thus, more than 50% of all children of color, yet only one in six white non-Hispanic children, resides in communities where child poverty surpasses 30% (Bruner, 2017). This data is critical when comparing communities for their larger effects on individual growth and development (Bruner, 2017). African American, Hispanic, or Native Americans predominately reside in these census tracts which comprise young children who are developing within a non-dominant culture community with much less financial capital and numerous concerns associated with meeting fundamental needs (Bruner, 2017). In these communities, it is essential that cultural reciprocity occurs and other attempts to promote and develop early childhood leadership along with service provisions from within these communities (Bruner, 2017). The norm for many young people in urban areas is that they frequently experience continual or chronic traumatic stress (Cohen et al., 2016). Examples of community level risk factors include poverty, lack of academic opportunity, residential segregation, lack of a built environment, poor social networks, lack of trust, high unemployment, high substance abuse/misuse, poor racial and intergroup relations, and poor health, educational, economic and social policies (Cohen et al., 2016). There are some places in the community where children live that create vulnerabilities to healthy development and shape the paths of their growth in profound ways. For instance, in extreme circumstances children who develop in hostile environments and relentless external brutality display the consequences of such assaults much more profoundly compared to adults (Cohen et al., 2016). These communities are described by physical as well as financial conditions that give rise to adversity; families are subjected to great levels of stress and consequently, ACEs in the household are more apt to surface (Cohen et al., 2016). While inherent human resources occur within all communities, pragmatically these resources are developed and realized in the context of the opportunities that exist within the "village." Realistically, the more troubled a community, the more the day-to-day toll of striving to survive and remain safe produces stress. The more society disinvests in select communities, the fewer reference points for success occur whereby children and their families can place genuine hopes for their own prospect of thriving during their life course. We must not only take an individually-based focus on services and underpinnings for young children and their families, there must also be investment in community-building endeavors to support and bolster its capacity to strengthen its children (Bruner, 2017).

Within the community, it is understandable that ACEs and poverty have a significant effect on school engagement and an array of health and well-being conditions over the life course (Travis, 2017). Osher and colleagues (2018) state that "schools are dynamic, multilevel, multilayered contexts for human development where teachers, peers, classrooms, public spaces and structures, culture, composition, policies, and student attributes influence each other" (p. 18). Importantly, schools have the capability of being created and organized in a manner that support individuals by affording a network of support and nurturing developmental relationships for students with their educators and fellow students (Osher et al., 2018). However, if the design and organization of schools do not promote environments for knowledge development, student- focused education, and cultural responsiveness, schools can in fact injure students in that moment and long-term (Osher et al., 2018). Of note, performance disparities among students have been explained by an environment of distrust, where students believe the school climate feels unfair and unsafe, with low expectations and bias (Travis, 2017). The lack of quality education at the community level impacts individual outcomes, for example literacy and the bond to schools (Lyles, Davis, Cohen, & Lester, 2017). Adverse experiences students encounter in school and in their communities can include dating abuse/intimate partner violence, bullying, peer fighting, gender-based sexual harassment, homophobic, racist and xenophobic abuse, and mass shootings (Osher et al.,

2018). Also, classroom climates typified by conflict are related to poor peer relations, enhanced aggression, and inferior outcomes academically and performance-based (Osher et al., 2018). Eventually, adverse experiences in school can bring about a cascade of deleterious educational and behavioral transactions that can steer children to pull back and become less driven, causing immense disparities in academic execution and accomplishment (Osher et al., 2018). This withdrawal can add to decreased attendance and poor grades in classes, disciplinary concerns (e.g., suspension, that may well result in dropout and school failure), and repeating grades (Osher et al., 2018). Exclusionary discipline affords an exemplar of school-generated adverse effects; utilization of exclusionary discipline promotes the experience of humiliation, student withdrawal, dropout, and arrests (Osher et al., 2018). Moreover, exclusionary discipline can adversely influence the learning, engagement, and feeling of safety of students who are not suspended (Osher et al., 2018). Consequently, both communities and schools can further the intergenerational transmission of adversity. Relevant to schools, they have the capacity to create as well as amplify risk (Osher et al., 2018).

What we learn from this information is that the accrual of community risk is one clear illustration of health inequities, the preventable, avoidable, and unjust differences in the incidence, prevalence, mortality, and affliction of ailments and other adverse health conditions (e.g., ACEs) that occur among particular population groups (Cohen et al., 2016). The provisions of such environments in communities stem from historical and existing policies, practices, and procedures as a role of government and other institutions (Cohen et al., 2016). Inequities in residential spaces, academics, health care, land use, criminal justice, community design, and labor force and economic development have contributed to substantial variations in community as well as individual opportunity and resources (Cohen et al., 2016). Regardless of how these inequities surface—purposeful and deliberate, unintentional, or neglectful, independently and cumulatively—they have aided in unfair disparities in health and safety (Cohen et al., 2016).

As health professionals who hold varied positions (e.g., practitioner, researcher, advocate, policy maker, administrator, or educator), we must seek to decide how we will draw upon the discoveries from ACEs research to optimize the health of individuals across the life course. We must appreciate early childhood adversity as broader than the particular ACEs indicator; these indicators have a place component. Looking outside of individual and family indicators of adversity is necessary to broaden our lens beyond individually-focused service responses, directed at certain adverse events and attempting to alleviate wounds that have already occurred. This action shifts in the direction of neighborhood-focused and community-building approaches (population health) intended to produce added resources.

In summary, communities are part of the village and social environment that can produce favorable or unfavorable contexts as well as display values and beliefs about what is acceptable for children's development. Racial and ethnic minorities have been disproportionately affected in a negative way. Understanding this landscape is critical to supporting transformation of all communities to enable individuals to live the best lives that they can.

Structural

Structural mechanisms (e.g., poverty, segregation, inequity, racism, gender discrimination, and systemic violence) that influence ACEs display the social layouts that place individuals and populations in harm's way (Montesanti & Thurston, 2015). Structural processes are created into the fabric of society comprising the political and financial organizations of our social world. Undoubtedly, these structures manufacture and uphold inequalities within and among dissimilar social groups in addition to ethnic, cultural, or other minority groups (Montesanti & Thurston, 2015). Accordingly, Sykes, Piquero, and Gioviano (2017) identify that neighborhood hardship focuses on the magnitude to which excessive poverty is directly located in specific locations—urban areas. Significantly, housing disadvantage and associated structural disorders such as family disruption, underemployment and unemployment, as well as inadequate schools are often situated largely in minority, but particularly in African American, areas in major cities (Sykes et al., 2017). Recognizing that these structural processes habitually go unimpeded since they are rendered invisible and can display themselves implicitly. This invisibility is maintained by power relations functioning from numerous points (West, 2014). Consequently, when intentionally examining these structures, we must investigate the *everydayness* of structures that foster ACEs from the perspective of multifaceted processes— historic, political, social, and economic (Montesanti & Thurston, 2015). Structural processes are expressed in unemployment, unequal access to goods, services like social support programs, and/or spaces, which impacts a range of determinants of health (Montesanti & Thurston, 2015). For example, structural macrosystem factors institutionalize practices, similar to public and private housing policy that furthers housing segregation which moderates accumulation of capital. Nevertheless, toxic structural macrosystem factors can be safeguarded by constructive factors, for instance healthy bonds to neighbors, feelings of belonging, and by wholesome microsystem contexts, such as progressive nourishing relationships with family members, educators, and peers (Osher et al., 2018).

In the United States, socially patterned variation is most dramatic for race (Umberson, 2017). Race is a structural system of inequality that systematically levies risks and stressors and undermines opportunities and resources for black Americans; structural conditions associated with segregation and discrimination subject black Americans to great levels of stress and limited resources (Umberson, 2017). Higher levels of stress related to racism and discrimination originate in childhood and remain throughout the life course, augmenting cumulative disadvantage in health over time (Umberson, 2017). This disadvantage is dramatically illustrated in increased race differences in exposure to ACEs, life expectancy, and mortality risk (Ellis & Dietz, 2017; Fink & Galea, 2015; Geronimus, Bound, & Colen 2011; McEwen & McEwen, 2017; Tomer, 2014; Umberson, 2017; Wade et al., 2014, 2015). West (2014) asserts that cultural racism is a tool of structural violence and is identified as:

> the systematic manner in which the white majority has established its primary cultural institutions (e.g., education, mass media and religion) to elevate and glorify European physical characteristics, character and achievement and to denigrate the physical characteristics, character and achievement of non-white people.
>
> *(p. 368)*

An expanded ACE variable, violence, is also pervasive especially among specific populations. Structural violence fuels the perpetuation of conditions that exacerbate ACEs and is increasingly recognized in population and public health as a major determinant of the dispersal and results of social and health inequities (Browne et al., 2016). Structural violence often alluded to as discrimination is the disadvantage and suffering resulting from the formation and continuation of structures, policies and institutional practices that are inherently unjust (Browne et al., 2016; West, 2014). While structural violence is often alluded to as discrimination, and cultural violence as prejudice, Galtung argues that formulating this sanitized language represents cultural violence itself (West, 2014). Respectively, cultural violence authorizes inequity, such as media and discourse and produces a shared consciousness of internalized and obvious oppression (West, 2014). These beliefs incorporate "the conscious and nonconscious view, attitudes, and actions that create everyday social realities" (West, 2014, p. 369). Given that systemic exclusion and hardship are fostered into routine social patterns and institutional processes, structural violence generates the conditions which nurture the production of health and social inequities (Browne et al., 2016). Also, since structural violence can be "static, insidious, silent, taken-for-granted, and hidden," it can cause people to believe that disparities in health and income, risks for exposure to ACEs, as well as good luck are the way things are (Browne et al., 2016, p. 545).

Sabo and colleagues (2014) find that immigrants of Hispanic origin encounter everyday violence and ACEs in varied areas including policy and militarization. Such adversity can depict structural racism, a form of cultural violence, as "the exploitive and oppressive social relationships that simultaneously define racial/ethnic groups and cause a system of inequalities that become embodied as racial/ethnic health inequities, invisible to its victims" (Sabo et al., 2014, p. 66). Galtung argues that it is exactly the exemplification of these social interactions that produce structural violence: "if there were reasons to believe that inequality, injustice, exploitation, penetration, fragmentation and marginalization were something given by nature, something forever beyond the power of man to counteract, then I would not speak of violence (as cited in West, 2014, p. 53)." The adversities encountered across the age spectrum for many Hispanics amount to everyday violence on the US-Mexico border; it is the discernible and violent display of structural racism and is the space where the arm of the state directly threatens the oppressed (Sabo et al., 2014). Institutionalized traditions of ethno-racial profiling enforced by immigration representatives are historically entrenched and deeply embedded at both the institutional and individual levels. Consequently, this operates to reproduce discrimination practices over time and at many levels (Sabo et al., 2014). Similarly, the health of Indigenous person's worldwide is formed by ordinary global colonial and neo-colonial forces with great resemblances in the colonizing processes as it relates to Indigenous individuals' experiences in many countries rendering these processes applicable internationally (Sabo et al., 2014). While some Indigenous communities have prospered in spite of colonial forces, enduring social inequities persist with harmful health effects for many Indigenous children, adolescents and adults (Browne et al., 2016). Colonialism is a social determinant of health and a trauma which impacts individuals across the life course (Czyzewski, 2011). It is important to understand how these processes have implications for ACEs and trauma experienced as an adult. Acknowledging the relationship between historical processes and its structurally oppressive forces and the link to present-day realities for children growing up is vital particularly while not losing sight of the numerous individual experiences that exist and the distinct contexts in which they were produced (Czyzewski, 2011). When a person is traumatized, authentic recognition is warranted since the dominant society does not allocate equal value to each person. However, the dominant society can be a resource to encourage just practices as well as to attest to the actuality of oppression and maltreatment giving these concepts social and political power. Clearly, intergenerational and historical trauma imparts specific consequences of colonial policies on individuals and conceivably entire communities (Czyzewski, 2011).

Present-day trauma of indigenous people in Canada is illustrated in that both the conception of reserve lands with resources insufficient for sustenance, and the trepidation of Indigenous children housed by the state, initially through residential schools and then to foster homes, have had deep harmful results over many generations (Browne et al., 2016). Likewise, in Australia, comparable efforts to assimilation were executed through the forced abstraction of children from Aboriginal and Torres Strait Islander communities (Browne et al., 2016). Throughout colonial contexts, these involuntary removals are frequently denoted as the stolen generation, and substantiation of the damaging health and social effects keeps accumulating (Browne et al., 2016). At present, the legacy of colonialism, systemic racism and other discriminatory practices promote the existing lack of employment opportunities, restricted access to quality education, insufficient affordable housing, and elevated levels of poverty faced by numerous Indigenous individuals in Canada, Australia, as well as other colonized countries worldwide (Browne et al., 2016).

While these structural mechanisms may well fall under the conceptualization of trauma and be used increasingly to apprise care delivered to individuals who are marginalized (i.e., excluded from significant engagement in social, economic, and political life) by social and structural inequities, we must remember that it encompasses more than traumatic events that have transpired in the past and more than just the psychological realm of a person's being (Browne et al., 2016). The effects of trauma must not be concealed as it relates to the effects of structural violence currently and we should not pathologize the effected person as a result of its impact on them (e.g., Indigenous people) (Browne et al., 2016). Accordingly, when applicable it is advised to use a decolonizing lens when examining issues of ACEs and trauma in relation to Indigenous or other colonized persons (Browne et al., 2016). Having a focus beyond the individual level and emphasis on the structural violence and the conditions that support it is critical (Browne et al., 2016). Importantly, Han (2017) acknowledges that "racism, poverty, violence in communities, as well as other structural inequities are inextricably linked with childhood trauma" (¶ 13). Central to transformation is making trauma visible and engaging communities in which trauma happens and understanding what makes it readily possible within existing structural dynamics. Unfortunately, discussions, policy and the broader media seldom make links between childhood trauma and enduring structural inequities (Han, 2017).

As health professionals, we need to realize that some Indigenous and colonized people may be survivors of numerous forms of violence with traumatic effects, while also experiencing current and continuing forms of violence (e.g., racial violence, bullying, and intimate partner violence) (Browne et al., 2016). As well, continued structural violence (systemic and structural racism and deep poverty) is also present (Browne et al., 2016). Modifying care, consequently, requires delivering comprehensive seamless care that concurrently attends to the many effects of related forms of violence (Browne et al., 2016). That said, health care providers have a critical role in diminishing suffering historically and ethically. The social determinants lens points out the necessity of integrating clinical care with endeavors to optimize a person's structural environment (Braveman & Gottlieb, 2014). Didactic and clinical education of health professionals in structural competency is needed; also, employing partnerships that start to tackle upstream structural factors (e.g., social cohesion, economic opportunity, racial disadvantage, and life satisfaction) is rather important. Significantly, health professionals can be important resources for local, state, and national policy makers on the fundamental issues of health equity for all people in their communities, including those encountering the greatest social impediments (Braveman & Gottlieb, 2014).

In summary, space matters greatly for young children, initially within the safety and security of their residential milieu, then their direct community environment, and ultimately the values and practices enforced through national policy. Specifically, attention to community environment and the interlaced matters of poverty, location, adversity, and race are integral to risks for exposure to ACEs and undesirable health outcomes. From a macro perspective, structural violence is central to the level of security, well-being, and happiness a person will experience across the life course. While structural violence is omnipresent, we know that individuals who are poor and from marginalized groups, especially racial minorities, experience its most damaging effects which also parallels higher ACEs scores (Wade, 2014, 2015; West, 2014). Health professionals must be sensitive to the fact that though direct violence is horrifying, its viciousness typically gains attention to some level depending on who it affects. However, the pernicious nature of structural violence is virtually always rendered invisible and is rooted in pervasive social structures, normalized by established institutions in our society.

PART III

Reducing ACEs

8

SOCIOECOLOGICAL MODEL

Individual and family influences

Primary prevention of ACEs across the life course should garner at least as much if not more prominence as responses to ACEs once they occur. The Vermont Department of Health (2014) insists, "(T)here isn't enough thought about prevention. So much of what we do is reactive…we are missing the boat on prevention" (p. 23). As Frederick Douglas states, "It's easier to build strong children than repair broken men" (Hanna-Attisha, 2017, p. 652). This necessitates full engagement of numerous systems within our society including evaluation of strategies implemented as well as attention in varied domains such as ontogenic, microsystem, exosystem and macrosystem. There are multiple biopsychosociocultural, political, and economic perspectives and interactive practices situated within and across these domains (Kim, 2017). An interactive process ensues in these varied domains, contexts, cultures as well as time periods; there are also numerous factors which may be predictive, protective, or indicative of heightened risk of ACEs as discussed in earlier chapter.

Moreover, science and evidence exist regarding how to prevent ACEs (Rantin, 2014). We need to be intentional with implementation of ways to place this learning into practice as well as to continue to assess and develop innovative learning about what works. Our goal should not only be primary prevention (i.e., intervene prior to something becoming a problem) of ACEs and protection of this generation of children, we must aim to build resilience and support them to thrive and live their best lives possible in order to strengthen the generation to come (Haynes et al., 2015). No single approach to ACE prevention exists and resolving the issue does not land in the purview of a single person, organization or state agency. Fundamentally, making prevention visible is requisite and in order for that to occur it is necessary to illustrate the context in which ACEs take place. While this chapter will specifically focus on the ontogenic and microsystem level factors to address prevention and protective factors which are associated with building resilience, Chapter 9 will highlight exosystem and macrosystem level elements of prevention and protection. It's important to keep in mind that a successful approach to prevention of ACEs requires an all-of-society approach (Metzler et al., 2017). Individual variables and familial factors can support and protect individuals across the life course as a result of personal resources. Buffers and supports need to be in position to aid parents who could otherwise be at risk of exposing their children to ACEs. For example, children are safer and maltreatment is less likely to take place when families are economically secure, healthy and flexible (Kim, 2017). Thus, protective factors buffer children from ACEs and resilience allows a dynamic system to resist or recover from momentous challenges that compromise its stability, viability, or development. The presence of these factors can lessen or eradicate risk within the microsystem. Next we will explore the concept of resilience, protective and prevention factors encompassed by the person, and subsequently microsystem level factors.

Resilience

> "Human resilience is about removing the barriers that hold people back in their freedom to act. It is also about enabling disadvantaged and excluded groups to express their concerns, to be heard and to be active agents in shaping their destiny."
>
> *(United Nations Development Programme (UNDP), 2014)*

An individual's wellbeing is affected to a great extent by the substantial freedoms within which the person lives as well as by their capability to react to and recover from adverse events (e.g., natural or human-made) (UNDP, 2014). Resilience is not an all-or-nothing characteristic since it encompasses a spectrum of qualities that can be acquired to varying degrees; it is a dynamic concept with a focus on bolstering any tactic to safeguarding and nourishing human development (Hornor, 2017). Resilience is characteristically described as "a pattern of positive adaptation in the context of past or present adversity" (Anthony, 2017, ¶ 2). However, a preferred definition by the authors is resiliency as protective or positive processes that diminish maladaptive outcomes when risks arise (Hornor, 2017). In fact, Rogers (2015) states that resilience is a protective factor, actually, many protective factors. As a protective factor it allows us to neutralize the risk factors that jeopardize our health. Anasuri (2016) states that resilience is not natural; it is a learned process that can be differentiated into two components—emergent resilience and minimal impact resilience. Emergent resilience is depicted as positive adjustment in the face of chronically occurring conditions, while minimal impact resilience is positive change across more insular, acute adverse events (Anasuri, 2016). Comprising more than a fixed individual trait, resilience is both a multifaceted phenomenon that consists of individual, relational, and contextual factors and it is not a permanent characteristic that a person embodies. In broad terms, resilience helps to make sure that state, community and global establishments operate to empower and protect people (UNDP, 2014). Human development involves eradicating the obstacles that prevent individuals from excelling in their autonomy to act.

Relevant then is assisting the underprivileged and disregarded to recognize their rights, to communicate their concerns freely, to be understood and to come to be active agents in forming their destiny (UNDP, 2014). Being able to possess the self-determination to live a life that an individual values and to manage their affairs effectively are also central components of human development that foster resilience. Importantly, individuals with inadequate core competences, such as education and health, are less adept at applying their agency to live lives they value. Moreover, to understand how resilience functions across the varied domains, a person's options may be limited or hampered by social impediments and other exclusionary practices; this can further implant social bias in public organizations and policies. However, responsive organizations and effective policy interventions can produce a sustainable dynamic to strengthen individual abilities and social conditions that improve human agency (i.e., making persons and societies more resilient). Education and investment, particularly for the extremely young, can prepare individuals to acclimate when an economic or natural disaster seizes their livelihood (UNDP, 2014).

An individual's developmental progression and changing life conditions can significantly modify resilience. While building resilience can allow a person to effectively cope with significant adversity at one stage in his or her life, they can respond negatively to other adversities at a future time. It is also important to make a distinction between resilience and thriving. Though day-to-day we often reflect on building resilience to support wellbeing, ultimately our goal should be to promote development beyond what is normal. Thus, resiliency is directly identified with adequacy whereas thriving is linked to excellence. When individuals thrive they often (a) feel progress or at least obtain achievement exceeding their functioning prior to encountering significant adversity, (b) have an active approach to achieving their goals, (c) have personal optimism and deliberate resolve that inspire personal agency beliefs, as well as (d) have a sense of vitality (aliveness).

When considering age across the life course, resilience in adolescence is a particularly complex process given the distinctive risk and prominent protective factors of this developmental stage, including enhanced hazard of destructive behavioral and emotional outcomes. These risks are intensified in adolescence due to vulnerabilities comprising rapid changes, strong desire for independence, and peer influences. Protective factors arise contextually and situationally, and therefore, could bring about dissimilar results. Moreover, protective factors that advantage one person in one context might not generate resilience in the same individual with other adverse factors or at a changed developmental stage (Kim, 2017). Accordingly, peer support may be considerably visible in the adolescent time period compared to other developmental stages attributable to higher influence of peers at this stage (Kim, 2017). Importantly, the more risks that an individual is exposed to, the less likely they are to experience protection or resilience. Ungar (2015) believes resilience, is less an indication of the person's ability to surmount life challenges but more related to the individual's informal and formal social networks that can aid in positive development under adversity. Consequently, caring connected environments are more vital to positive acclimatization to challenges than the presence of a particular inherent genetic trait or characteristic (Ungar, 2015).

It is important for health professionals to understand building resilience. The lens used to understand this concept can inform what professionals may consider to be maladaptive yet could be considered protective for a specific individual. In our present-day diverse society, it is increasingly essential to distinguish the variation in adaptation, and offer culturally sensitive supports. Resilience inherently advances early intervention in contrast to treatment, as in situations when health professionals are seeking issues to resolve. Hence, encouraging resilience is not just pursuing those who are demonstrating challenging symptoms, which may unsuccessfully recognize children who are enduring adverse circumstances. Instead, resilience is continuing to develop the strengths and resources each individual possesses and is capable of accessing within their environment (Kim, 2017). A conceivable concern with resilience is the likelihood for it to be comprehended as a personal trait (i.e. resiliency), and intrinsically, a person's responsibility for attaining the skills essential to be successful. This is expressly problematical with at-risk children and youth, who confront environmental adversity that stretches far beyond *trying harder* (Kim, 2017). Consequently, by delineating resilience within a social-ecological context, the responsibility is on the broader community to advance resilience (Ungar, 2015). Also, in order to enhance resilience, it is important to comprehend that people are "embedded in families, families in organizations and communities, and communities in societies and cultures" (Rogers, 2015, p. 59). This too is a logical scenario as the gains from positive adaptation, or the failures of maladjustment, will be experienced in the broader community (Kim, 2017). The following section will highlight prevention efforts which enable action to be taken to build resilience and to prevent problems before they occur or processes to intervene earlier in the process. While treatment for ACEs is laudable, we must recognize an important statement by Dr. George Albee, "No epidemic has ever been resolved by paying attention to the treatment of the affected individual" (Lyles, Davis, Cohen, & Lester, 2017, p. 8).

Ontogenic

Ontogenic factors, the innermost domain, represent the personal history (i.e., internal factors) that shape the person's behavior, relationships, and developmental adaptation. Both internal and external resources serve as protective factors that help to prevent ACEs such as neurobiology/ genetic variation, personality traits such as temperament, social competence, high ego control and self-esteem, elevated internal locus of control, external attributions of blame, ascription of success to own efforts as well as favorable relationship capabilities, and age (National Academy of Sciences, 2014). Moreover, intelligence or cognitive ability is perceived as a personal protective factor (National Academy of Sciences, 2014). Additionally, an individual having knowledge that they can handle a situation, confidence in one's own abilities, morals and values that demonstrate understanding how one's behavior affects others, coping, including the ability to focus on decisions as well as planning, all help with prevention of adversity from an ontogenic perspective (Hornor, 2017). Developmental strengths epitomize internal (e.g., positive values) and external (e.g., boundaries and expectations) resources that play a part in an individual's ability to thrive. Promotive factors (e.g., labeled assets or resources) are those related to better outcomes and may contribute to mediating positive outcomes across more than one domain; this is briefly highlighted in ontogenic prevention through protection examples below.

Neurobiology/ genetic variation. Fostering a healthy brain is vitally important. Early human development is a complex and dynamic process between nature and nurture or genes and the environment. Thus, genes respond to the environment, and the environment alters one's genetic blueprint. Accordingly, clear prevention that serves to protect individuals is being immersed in largely a wholesome environment. This is crucial as the environment modifies expression of genes (e.g., gene variants or phenotype); genes can be turned on and off via the epigenetic process. As noted in an earlier chapter, these experiences assign a chemical signature (i.e., epigenetic mark) modifying genetic expression short of modifying the DNA sequence; these changes can be temporary however some endure (UNDP, 2014). No one gene or gene variation marks resilience, nevertheless genetic factors perform an essential role in governing how an individual responds to adversity. Optimization of prenatal and early-life experience along with genetics contributes to the person's neurobiology and spectrum of resilience as well as minimization of adversity (Rogers, 2015).

Age. Children maneuver within a very delicate stage of life. Notwithstanding other potential issues, childhood is a vulnerable stage of life requiring safeguarding to prevent ACEs given the lack of complete control of their lives. Accordingly, building resilience can be challenged since this age group commonly fears independence, responsibility and failure, and dislikes to exercise choice which contrasts against resilience (Anasuri, 2016). However, resilience is pronounced in children when their lives are fruitful in resources—having strong sense of self-concept, caring parent-child relationships, and friendly and warm relationships with teachers. Preventing children from living in environments under chronic stresses is critical; protecting the child by providing them with safe, stable, and loving environments to optimize positive psychological and emotional resources as well as basic physical necessities promotes prevention of ACEs and resilience. Research has shown that championing for a child's physical, cognitive, social, and emotional development sets them on a healthy path (Biglan et al., 2017; National Academy of Sciences, 2014). For instance, children with strong social competency, such as identifying feelings in themselves and others, effectively dealing with their thoughts and emotions, and working out interpersonal problems, are more apt to attend college later in life or hold a full-time employment, and are less prone to abuse drugs or alcohol or commit a crime (National Academy of Sciences, 2014). Adolescents have greater development and life experience than children physically, emotionally, and psychologically. This too brings many challenges; therefore gaining the necessary tools to best manage adversity (e.g. bullying, relational aggression) can help prevent ACEs. Social pressures and parental conflict can be very pronounced during this developmental stage. Protective factors including problem-solving, internal locus of control, strong sense of independence, higher self-esteem, supportive family systems, and social engagement can help to mitigate ACEs and build resilience. Differing demographics can inform risk for ACEs such as the experience of discrimination. Therefore, building positive identity formation especially racial identity is keenly important in the US. Often, it is early in life where viewpoints are constructed that influence how a person feels about themselves; the goal is for the individual to feel good about himself/herself (self-esteem, self-worth, self-regard) and what they can achieve (self-efficacy). When formed early in life, these perspectives tend to evolve throughout development having significant effects during adolescents (Skousen, n.d.). Resiliency theory recognizes the following factors align more with high ACEs and often low resiliency— low socioeconomic status, dropping out of school, participation in violent activities, recent divorce, neglect, poverty, teenage pregnancy, and teenage parenthood. Accordingly, optimizing parental, teacher, and friend support is important. For adolescents and young adults, events stemming from their daily lives can produce intense emotions that are often challenging for them to control, as a result effective coping strategies are paramount (e.g., listening to music, therapeutic engagement with a behavioral health professional, and healthy social interactions) (Anasuri, 2016).

Social competence/social resources/ relational skills. The ability to effectively connect and interact well with others serves as a useful skill. Being able to attain tangible support in times of need is also a valuable asset that mitigates exposure to ACEs. Additionally, protective factors include involvement in positive activities especially with peers. Thus, building resilience through relational skills optimizes an individual's well-being by having: (a) an ability to form positive bonds and connections (e.g., social competence, being caring, forming positive attachments and prosocial relationships); (b) favorable interpersonal proficiencies such as communication skills, conflict resolution skills, and self-efficacy in conflict situations; and (c) self-regulation (e.g., managing or controlling one's emotions and behavior, self-mastery, and anger management) (Rogers, 2015).

Problem solving. An ultimate preventive measure for ACEs is when an individual has an ability to proactively respond and address challenging situations as well as plan for life in a manner that averts adversity. Elevated problem-solving skills enable heightened self-efficacy in discordant situations, decision-making skills, planning skills, adaptive functioning skills and task-oriented coping skills (Brodowski & Fischman, 2013).

Microsystem

Microsystem denotes the ecologies most proximal to the child, including the family and peer relationships and those systems that are intimately related to the family (e.g., family functioning and school environments) (Hornor, 2017). Family-level protective factors such as having a safe, stable, nurturing family are integral to healthy child development and promotion of well-being across the life course. Additional prevention strategies that can lead to protection include healthy connections that occur with parents, siblings, older adults, faith or spiritual community, school and peers. Moreover, being able to work as a team or serving others in meaningful ways also helps to promote resilience and minimize adversity. Micro-level processes that further serve as protective mechanisms include improving the culture, attitudes, and relations in communities, schools, peer groups, and families by focusing on fostering communication skills and values that promote positive developmental processes, such as parenting classes, antibullying policies and programs, and drug education programs (Hornor, 2017). These protective mechanisms are frequently designed for children's relationships, specifically bolstering relationships with parents, siblings, and other relatives and peers. This is key, since healthy relationships build resilience and diminish exposure to ACEs (Hornor, 2017).

When parents engage children through reading, they create healthy bonds and have improved cognitive development giving children essential means for healthy, fruitful lives. Early childhood is a propitious stage to promote equity, given that unaddressed disparities throughout the primary years produce exaggerated problems introducing greater levels of adversity and also extending social, academic, and economic gaps (Davis, Costigan, & Schubert, 2017). Importantly, depending on context, all common protective factors (e.g., family) do not transcend every situation and therefore protective factors are situational with context and time driven. For example, a young girl who is sexually abused by family may have to be removed and placed in foster care. While family may not be protective in this circumstance, peer affects and warmth received from school undoubtedly can serve as a positive future orientation (National Academy of Sciences, 2014). Non-family members who have relationships with individuals can deter ACEs by having them exposed to understanding teachers as well as caring relationships with peers, work colleagues, and religious personnel (National Academy of Sciences, 2014). Optimizing levels of social cohesion is favorable towards mitigating exposure to ACEs such as positive family socioeconomic factors (income or education) and demographic factors (family structure), ideological factors (shared values among those close to the person) as well as the accessibility of an enviable social support system (formal and informal).

Given the relevance of families in serving as a protective mechanism against ACEs, the following section will highlight some programs that serve to promote resilience:

■ *Strengthening Families Initiative (SFI)*

SFI, a preventive intervention to mobilize protective factors around all families in a community, was developed by the *Center for the Study of Social Policy* (van Dijken, Stams, & Winter, 2016). The goal of SFI is to influence parent behavior by employing an existing service delivery system and promoting five protective factors that serve to increase the well-being of children and their families. The specific protective factors targeted are: (a) parental resilience, (b) social connections, (c) knowledge of parenting and child development, (d) concrete support in times of need, and (e) social and emotional competence of children. In order to effectively support families with increasing protective factors and to support parents in detecting signs of stress at an early phase, child and family serving professionals also receive training to successfully execute their role. Specific sectors that implement SFI include early childhood home visiting, child welfare, as well as child abuse and neglect prevention and family support. Neighborhood processes are only addressed via the social connections factor. Actions supporting the social connections factor are built on the supposition that parents with a high level of social capital (e.g., a system of emotionally caring helpful friends, family and neighbors) have healthier relationships with their children. Furthermore, designing opportunities for parents to convene, in schools, faith-based establishments or other locations, can inspire secluded parents to solicit help. This belief is founded on study findings showing that social disorganization was the central factor that accounted for why dissimilar neighborhoods with comparable socioeconomic profiles had dissimilar rates of ACEs; the chief dissimilarity was their level of social capital (van Dijken et al., 2016).

Website: https://www.cssp.org/young-children-their-families/strengtheningfamilies/about

■ *The Incredible Years© Program*

This program aims to bolster parenting competencies including monitoring, positive discipline, and confidence. Additional emphasis is placed on nurturing parents' participation in children's school experiences with the intention of fostering children's educational, social, and emotional competencies and reducing behavioral concerns. Parents, teachers, and children ages 3–12 are the primary target group for this program. The program is carried out in a community agency, outpatient health center, or school setting typically in groups of 12–16 parents or groups of 6 children. Time commitment is 12–14 weeks for the Basic Parent Training program while it is 18–22 weeks for the Child Training Program. Website: www.incredibleyears.com

■ *Nurturing Parenting Programs®*

This program promotes parenting skills and prevents recidivism in families receiving social services. It also focuses on bolstering parent-teenager relations, decision making skills, and stopping the intergenerational cycle of child abuse. Parents of children aged from birth to 18 years old are engaged in this program in groups of 8–12 adults. Children meet in a separate group. This 12 to 48-week program is provided in birth family homes, community organizations, departments of social services and behavioral health, parent education programs, prisons, residential care facilities, as well as schools. Website: www.nurturingparenting.com

■ Triple P-Positive Parenting Program

This program strives to foster behavioral, emotional, and developmental well-being in children by strengthening the knowledge, skills, and confidence of parents. Parents and caregivers of children aged from birth to 16 years meet in groups of 10–12; children and adolescents from birth to age 16 are also engaged. The program is carried out in adoptive, birth, family, and foster homes; community organizations; hospitals and ambulatory health centers; residential care facilities; as well as schools. Website: www.TripleP-America.com

Schools, another important proximal entity which children occupy, can provide opportunity and enhance their quality of life. Capatosto (2015) argues that it is important for schools to: (a) focus on empowering students versus adversely placing focus on a child's behavior in a vacuum, (b) be attentive to the difficulties a student may confront and demonstrate effort to produce a milieu that permits them to thrive to the greatest degree possible, (c) promote goal orientation and enhance student safety in their learning environment, (d) endorse student learning through positive communication and emotional literacy in order to form rapport and encourage students to make positive behavior choices, and (e) use a strengths-based orientation to inform practices to promote student achievement. Additional strategies that promote resilience include embracing positive ethnic, racial, and intergroup relations; demonstrating respect for diversity and an emphasis on equity; and promoting healthy norms and expectations (Lyles et al., 2017).

Schools with an endeavor to transform their climate to a more nurturing environment for children often focus on social–emotional learning. According to the Organization for Economic Co-operation and Development in Biglan, Van Ryzin, and Hawkins (2017), the

TABLE 8.1 Other Programs that Support Prevention and Promote Healthy Development of Individuals

Name of Program	Link to additional information
Blueprints for Healthy Youth Development	https://www.colorado.edu/cspv/blueprints/
Child Trends What Works	http://www.childtrends.org/what-works/
Commissioning Toolkit of Parenting Programs – United Kingdom	http://webarchive.nationalarchives.gov.uk/20121031032820/https://www.education.gov.uk/publications/eOrderingDownload/Commissioning_Toolkit_user_guide.pdf
What Works Wisconsin: Evidence-Based Parenting Program Directory	https://fyi.uwex.edu/whatworkswisconsin/files/2014/04/whatworks_08.pdf
Promising Practices Network on Children, Families and Communities	http://www.promisingpractices.net/programs.asp
SafeCare	http://www.marcus.org/treatment/safecare.html
Staying Connected With Your Teen®	www.channing-bete.com/prevention-programs/staying-connected-w-your-teen/
STEP (Systematic Training for Effective Parenting)	www.parentingeducation.com
Family Check-Up (FCU)	https://homvee.acf.hhs.gov/Model/1/Family-Check-Up-For-Children-In-Brief/9
Nurse-Family Partnership	https://www.nursefamilypartnership.org/about/
Problem Solving Skills Training (PSST)	http://www.cebc4cw.org/program/problem-solving-skills-training/

United States ranks at the bottom among 32 high-resource countries in social–emotional learning in schools. However, programs that foster social–emotional learning can offer precise education in positive social interactions and effective problem solving thereby reducing problem behavior and enhancing academic achievement (Biglan et al., 2017).

The Good Behavior Game by Kellam et al. (2011) establishes a nurturing school environment by using a teaching strategy that functions on a philosophical perspective of social reinforcement of on-task and prosocial behavior. Children in Good Behavior Game classrooms are taught to restrain urges to act with aggression, disruption, and off-task behavior (Biglan et al., 2017). They become skilled at regulating emotions and examining their classmates behavior in a game-like setting. Moreover, Good Behavior Game and associated group or team-based instructional methods, for example, cooperative learning underscore the formation of positive interdependence in classrooms; this indicates that persons reach their goals when others they are working with also attain theirs. Accordingly, when implementing positive interdependence, within-group peer interaction, which formerly could have been indifferent or keenly aggressive, is more inclined to encourage the success of others via communal support and resource sharing. Such positive social interactions sequentially heighten interpersonal appeal and acceptance, encourage development of additional friendships, and, in a scholastic context, stimulate educational engagement and attainment. In effect, Bierman (2004) proposes that improvements in social skills only lack adequacy for decreasing social isolation and rejection; rather, positive interdependence is mandatory to stimulate youth to reconsider preceding assumptions concerning the social desirability of others.

Haynes and colleagues (2015) also endorse actions that can be taken to prevent ACEs in school and promote building resilience. Children and other students across the life course should gain age appropriate knowledge and awareness within curriculum about healthy child development as well as ACEs and associated implications, schools should optimize opportunities provided by non-teaching activities (e.g., school trips or break times) for school personnel (teachers, nurses, or counselors) to foster positive relationships with the students in their care. For example, in the United Kingdom, as part of the government's Healthy Child Programme, school nurses have accountability for children aged between 5 and 19. They are responsible for a variety of activities that support relationship-building, including offering advice, education and support, along with medical treatments (Haynes et al., 2015).

Finally, Bielenberg et al. (2015) highlighted an important program that inspires resilience through its Compassionate Schools initiative created by the Washington Office of Superintendent of Public Instruction. This program affords training, guidance, referral, and technical assistance to schools wanting to implement its infrastructure which advantages all students present. It also offers assistance to students who may be exposed to stress and trauma in their lives. Compassionate schools embody caring classrooms and cultivate compassionate attitudes of their school staff to facilitate student engagement and learning by crafting a healthy climate and culture within the school. Relevant principles of a compassionate school include:

a   Address culture and climate in the school and community
b   Educate and support all staff concerning trauma and learning
c   Inspire and support open and regular communication for all
d   Create a strengths-based style in working with students and peer

e   Make sure that discipline policies are compassionate and effective emphasizing their restorative nature
f   Integrate compassionate policies into school development planning
g   Deliver tiered support for the entire student body based on what they need
h   Produce flexible accommodations for different learners
i   Afford access, voice, and ownership for school employees, students and community
j   Employ data to both detect vulnerable students and establish outcomes and tactics for continuous quality improvement.

(Bielenberg et al., 2015)

In summary, domains used in the ecological model provide a useful framework to understand the way in which a combination of levels (e.g., ontogenic, microsystem, macrosystem, and exosystem) inform how prevention can lead to protection of individuals from ACEs. Building resilience is an active intentional process that is impacted by context and time. Varied strategies to build resilience are beneficial such as relational and emotional resilience arising from secure attachment with and affection from a parent, caregiver, or caring adult (protective factors); behavioral resilience stemming from the formation of healthy habits of focusing, persistence, endurance, and task completion; cognitive competence which occurs from learning strategies to promote positive thinking and building cognitive resilience; and learning how to develop and access ecological resources such as culturally and situationally appropriate coping responses and problem-solving skills.

Ecological approaches for cultivating resilience have much to offer with the ontogenic and micro-level system, given the focus on how individuals and their most proximal contacts and the environments interact together to create different opportunities. In particular, it is important to make more visible the ways in which contexts restrict or magnify the range of options children are able to attain and the subsequent opportunities that they will see they really have available to them at various points in time. Thus, individuals and relationships come together to produce opportunities for change; broader domains of support hold resources that others (e.g., vulnerable/marginalized individuals) need in order to construct opportunities for positive well-being. It is this realization that is embodied within an

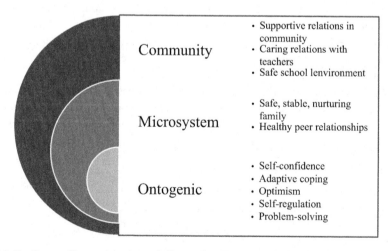

FIGURE 8.1 Resilience: Prevention through Protection Factors

ecological understanding of resilience however we only addressed the first two layers in this chapter. The next two layers (macrosystem and exosystem) will be discussed in Chapter 9. The processes that permit resilience to potentiate favorable outcomes are complex and entail a focus that progresses beyond attention to a specific factor or a small quantity of factors. As we will explore next, a broad-based prevention effort towards resilience requires exploration of resources, characteristics, and processes which are positioned in a variety of spaces from the individual (ontogenic level) through to the structural level.

9

SOCIOECOLOGICAL MODEL

Context and cultural influences

Resilience is an influential process where "meanings and practices [...] are always embedded in larger social, economic and political contexts" (Kovacic, 2015, p. 59). Understanding prevention through protection at these more distal systems which influence the individual indirectly allows us to view more holistically how these factors (e.g. economic and political systems) shape a person's health and resources for resilience. The interrelationships between both proximal (e.g. social and physical environments an individual inhabits) and distal environments (e.g., settings removed from the individual's direct environment) are just as powerful in individual development and resilience as any distinct event taking place in one's environment (Kovacic, 2015). Interestingly, the environments that affect behavior become progressively complex and distal as the individual ages (Botha, 2014). Environments or systems are presumed to be self-regulatory and have to uphold their own performance while acclimating to the demands of the context in which they occur (Botha, 2014). This is a shared process to facilitate the individual and environment to experience reciprocal transformation (Botha, 2014). While the individuals' functioning is being informed by their experiences, indicating that patterns of adjustment can be altered by environmental changes, environmental structures have diverse meanings and influences for distinct individuals thanks to their unique qualities; accordingly, their response to these experiences will be unique (Botha, 2014). Consequently, what each of us recognize, disregard, seek out or produce in our environments can amass to our advantage or disadvantage (Botha, 2014). Societies have the capability to expedite access to resources and support people and their families when subjected to life challenges. Preferably, being proactive with optimizing the well-being of individuals across the life course should be a shared goal nationally and globally.

Florin and Linkov (2016) state that by implementing strength-based approaches to how we function in society, essentially a proactive not reactive stance is taken thereby advocating for prevention of problems prior to them arising. Individuals can acquire numerous skills to contend with life by gaining a deep understanding of human factors, the built environment, and the natural environment and how they interact. However, myopic efforts limit reduction or elimination of risk to assure an optimal quality of life. Taking a broader perspective to understand how distal systems must focus on more than primarily preventing threats and risks is important but we also must produce policies that support the population to thrive in life. Understanding and fostering resilience needs to be a strategic societal priority that surely is concerned with more than the management of risk. Assuring that the communities and systems not only traverse recognized and unidentified risks of ACEs and other adversities, but become resilient and more thriving while transiting risky waters of life (Florin & Linkov, 2016).

In this section we will examine these more distal systems—exosystem and macrosystem. That said, implications for the community such as the workplace, medical settings, legal and educational system, as well as broader cultural factors dealing with policy will be discussed.

Exosystem

Communities and service agencies are viewed as the exo-level which is described as the space where individuals do not participate actively, nevertheless it influences their immediate environment. A resilient community is perceived as managing well all together and learning from challenging circumstances. These types of communities have resources and structures prepared to assist with transforming the environment through intentional efforts and collective action. For a child, this may well involve exchanges between parents/guardians, friends, and educators, and the family physician. The extent that these entities communicate with each other and have shared interests is a gauge of the child's ability to thrive. Additionally, a child may not interact directly with the parents' workplace; however it has a large effect on them. In fact, this may have negative effects on the child if his/her parents are unable to pay the rent, mortgage, purchase groceries, or if the workplace extends hours of the parent. These longer hours will influence parental behaviors and emotional capacity and parent-child interactions when they get home.

Moreover, the beliefs, values, and opportunities parents encounter at work, for instance regarding their autonomy or dependency, is what they often carry home and in effect require the same from their children (Lundberg & Wuermli, 2012). Accordingly, parents who were mostly submissive at work have a propensity to subdue their children. This element may assist with elucidating intergenerational transmission of values. Also, parental workplace schedule flexibility and supervisor support are related to greater parental warmth (Lawson et al., 2016). Given that workplace policies and practices can clearly affect the health and well-being of employees (e.g., parents of children) along with their work organizations, parents' workplaces are germane settings that have an effect on their child's development and adjustment (Lawson et al., 2016). What is more, since 88% of US families with dependent children normally have at least one working parent, these parents' workplaces have significant implications for a child's welfare and resilient-related resources (Lawson et al., 2016).

Regarding parental workplace, a key goal should be to foster prevention through protection by promoting equal opportunity to employees and emboldening an environment of equity, diversity, inclusion and positive growth and collaboration. Championing for holistic employee and parental development, while striving for a healthy work-life balance, enables numerous paths to realize optimal levels of wellness. For instance, workplaces can construct relaxation or comfort rooms where employees can take time-outs as needed, health and fitness programs can engage personnel, arts and creativity options can be made available, and opportunities to undertake meaningful roles for social impact can be mobilized in the work setting. Moreover, economic upsets can have a huge effect on exosystems, influencing not just the workplaces of parents but similarly the conditions of those who are not working. Some functions of work including how one organizes their day, earnings, and social status can be affected (Lundberg & Wuermli, 2012).

Similarly, educational districts and legal systems are part of the exosystem and can substantially influence fostering resilience. Accordingly, a state's department of education has an indirect influence on many aspects regarding resilience of children such as the quality of personnel students are exposed to including their credentialing requirements, position expectations, and program funding allotted to support nurturing students. As well, the education system such as board of directors of a health sciences university influences the type of training health care professionals obtain (e.g., ACE screening). Another system that can affect screening is the legal system. Health care professionals in medical settings may not screen due to uncertainty regarding mandatory reporting and apprehension about having suitable documentation when communicating with individuals in the legal system. Even when we look across the life course, Bruder (2013) states that all medical schools and residency programs are compelled to attend to trauma such as domestic violence. However, lack of training and education on recognizing and supporting those wounded by intimate partner violence is commonly described as an impediment to screening. Importantly, prevention through protection upholds the need to train routinely on these topics regardless of location of residency. Protocols set forth by systems and organizations can drive medical settings to implement measures that support health care professionals to routinely screen for intimate partner violence (Bruder, 2013). Educating health professionals on state-specific laws including legal parameters around disclosures would affect the ability to provide private and confidential care and support the safety and well-being of individuals.

Another important consideration related to the exosystem and educational system is socioeconomic status (SES); SES is directly associated with the educational system that a child is affiliated with—private versus public education—and conceivably influences the educational experiences individuals have as well as the educational messages they receive. Typically, an individual residing in a school district that adequately services the needs of their children is practically always governed by SES and districts with leading services characteristically have a higher SES population. There are ways in which these traditional circumstances hamper the growth of a child who comes from a low SES background. This occurs when powerful individuals in the organizations embedded in the exosystem produce critical decisions concerning policies, funding, and practices without regard for and collaboration with the professionals and populations who are directly affected by pertinent matters of interest. To promote prevention through protection educational systems should push for equitable means to support children and families to thrive. They will need to increase financial resources for health, human services, and education mainly for institutions and professionals that intercede in the lives of children and families that are devastated by perilous conditions of living with limited resources. Increased economic resources also need to be directed at prevention of behavioral health difficulties and socioeconomic concerns that impede personal and family resilience (Turner, 2009). Finally, engagement of key sponsors and persons within the target population is needed in policy formation, practical application processes, and funding rulings consisting of direct service workers, program executives, and families (Turner, 2009).

As part of the exosystem, medical settings are influential on a person due to decision-making by medical boards, the family's insurance company, and policies such as care

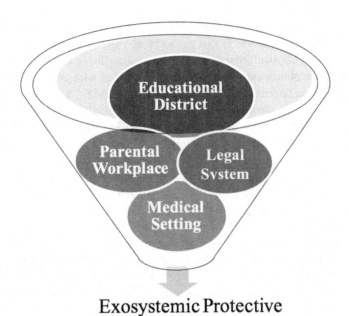

**Exosystemic Protective
Factors**

FIGURE 9.1 Examples of Exosystemic Protective Factors that Promote Resilience

delivered in a patient-and family-centered manner and hospital funding. These entities affect a child's medical care along with the family's experience of care. More specifically, the readiness of the health care system similarly has an effect on both the training received in addition to the structure of the health care setting at the exo-level. As an example, counseling and family therapists' training offers the skills desirable to effectively communicate within a medical setting and attend to emotional needs of personnel in addition to family. However, the structure of each health care setting impacts when, how, and why counseling and family therapists are welcomed onto the health care team. Another illustration that can foster prevention through protection is when a medical setting is attentive to care of the whole person and delivers inclusive care by offering ease of access to both physiological, mental health, and spiritual care along with services that optimize partnering in meaningful ways with individuals receiving their services. Imagine a systemic impediment of enforcing English-only language laws for an Argentinian American individual whose language of comfort is Spanish (Barrera, 2008). This impediment also makes it more challenging for Latinos who only speak English marginally to access mental health care. What's more, because mental health services are often not colocated or integrated into the same settings as traditional medical care or offer health information in their preferred language, individuals may become disheartened and ultimately not receive the mental health care needed (Barrera, 2008).

Regarding prevention, medical settings can offer protection by reducing the likelihood of maladaptive outcomes under conditions of risk from ACEs through implementation of universal ACE Screening across the life course. As noted in earlier chapters, ACEs are indicative of our social reality; however, those exposed to greater life challenges with fewer resources are impacted to a greater extent. As noted by Fallot and Harris (2009), "the experience of trauma is simply not the rare exception we once considered it" (p. 1). It is part and parcel of our social reality. Health professionals within the exosystem often assist children by supplying parents with knowledge and resources that can enhance their children's welfare. Screening to assess for family conditions that do not promote wholesome living conditions (e.g., unsafe or maladaptive) affords mobilization of supports that are aligned with desirable outcomes. Universal ACE and trauma screening can educate many about ACEs, its associated implications, and prevention efforts and identify at-risk or existing individuals who have been wounded. In essence, this delivers an element of primary prevention through universal exposure of individuals seeking medical care to questions and education on these related areas of adversity.

General practitioners tend to care for families over many years and connect with multiple members of the same families which can allow for a holistic view of a family, especially when a member of the family has long-term health needs (Haynes et al., 2015). They frequently garner respect from individuals and families they serve and should have culturally proficient skills to coach and offer advice on how to promote well-being (Haynes et al., 2015). For example, in the United Kingdom, included in the government's Healthy Child Programme, school nurses are responsible for children 5 through 19 years old. Being able to form meaningful relationships with the same youth over time allows nurses to see which protective factors can be strengthened and employed as drivers of change, consequently precluding needless, negative trajectories for children they connect with (Haynes et al., 2015).

To support building resilience and offering nurturing relationships to individuals by health professionals, de Zulueta (2016) states that the work experience of health care personnel is vital to their own and their clients' well-being, along with the general culture of the health care workplace. This underscores the need for providing personnel well-being structures and practices. Quite often, health professionals are exposed to elevated levels of negative emotions in taxing environments and must be adept in emotional regulation and adaptive approaches to manage oneself (de Zulueta, 2016). While training and education regarding these elements will benefit health professionals, the organizational environment in which they are embedded must be conducive to promote delivery of compassionate care to individuals across the life course. No amount of resilience by the health professional will weather obstructive, unsupportive, or toxic organizational cultures, especially if the champions who raise their voice are silenced or compelled to depart from the organization (de Zulueta, 2016). With that said, prevention through protection for health personnel would include:

- Allowing health personnel to come together and have discourse around challenging emotional and social matters in caring for clients. This supports enhancing staff well-being and morale.
- Implementing appreciative inquiry which fosters strength and produces lexis of hope, inspiring, and stimulating people to change. Appreciative inquiry is known to galvanize community building with widespread use of storytelling.
- Recognizing that appreciative inquiry and appreciative storytelling along with mindfulness education has surfaced as valuable to health professionals' well-being, increasing empathy, reducing burnout, and boosting patient satisfaction.
- Utilizing mindfulness meditation and compassionate mind training can enhance awareness to suffering and psychological litheness, heighten patient-centered value directed care, and foster self-compassion and emotional resilience.

(de Zulueta, 2015)

Ultimately, health professionals need to feel both safe in their organizational context and emboldened to show attentive kindness; as well, being in sync with their own needs and those of their clients is important along with having the resources and capability to take proper steps to ease distress. Equally important is for health personnel to build resilience for their clients by acknowledging their humanity and uniqueness (de Zulueta, 2015).

Macrosystem

Macrosystem consists of the politics, beliefs, relative freedoms permitted by the national government, the economy, wars, colonialism, and customs that characterize the cultural fabric of the individuals' society. This is the largest and most distant group of people and structures/organizations from developing individuals however it has great influence over him/her; it dictates children's place in society. Each community has an identifiable cultural history that comprises different traditional practices, rituals and beliefs regarding children. These macro-level elements can also affect resilience either favorably or negatively. Macrosystem factors, for example, type of government, media, cultural preferences and ideals and religions have a strong operational presence in the expectations, values and knowledge that people and local families in communities bring to bear day-to-day, especially in their memories and know-how; this can assist with the development of resilience (Boon et al., 2012). Notably, the macrosystem is the most invisible, even with its significant effect on people's lives. It affects social policies and services which regulate other layers (micro and exo), as well as the quality of a person's everyday life. This is directly linked with the ideologies and social institutions that characterize a specific culture or subculture along with laws, values and traditions of a society. Furthermore, the macro-level greatly impacts the predominant economic and political systems and popular discourses that establish the meaning a person ascribes to their roles and activities (Boon et al., 2012). That said, an individual's development and resources for resilience cannot be appreciated apart from their distinctive sociopolitical, historical and ideological conditions. Any ontogenic element, microsystem, or exosystem is a manifestation of the macrosystem; substantial resemblances transpire in the systems of any particular culture.

On a macro-level, endorsing prevention through protection requires contextual factors that foster a child's capability to excel, for instance, academically which is one of the most cost-effective ways of decreasing poverty and stimulating economic progress and success of a nation. On a macro-level, cultural beliefs and social policies overseeing entrée to economic, housing, scholastic and other opportunities, may exert a harmful effect on proximal processes, intensifying the effect of poverty on our most vulnerable—our children. To prevent ACEs we must also keep in mind that the intricate nature of the etiology of ACEs prevails beyond the person, the family, as well as the community where it is inextricably entwined; people develop linking the personal, interpersonal and socio-cultural factors and processes—the blueprint of the society. Thus, cultural principles, belief systems, societal structures, gender role socializations as well as society's views toward ACEs affect childhood development (Kovacic, 2015).

Taking the aforementioned information into consideration, it is apparent that there is an important link between external protective processes embedded on various societal levels, including families, schools, communities and a state, and individual coping and resilience (Kovacic, 2015). This is not surprising since protective factors are nurtured by societies and cultures though socio-political transformations have significant implications for these protectors. External protective factors (resources) promote significantly, for instance, youth resilience. A link between macrosystem factors (e.g. state and political ideologies) and other systemic and environmental levels of society has to be considered when examining what kind of resources are available for youth in these locations. Social policies and social values control how these resources are allocated and also navigated by young people. More specifically, Aiello, Tesi, Pratto, and Pierro (2017) identify that dominant groups' social values and policies monopolize social, political, and economical resources over marginalized populations. A clear example targeting the population level that can have the greatest individual and societal impact is supplying adequate salaries for people; however currently dominant groups in power refuse to pass legislation and policy to reduce resource disparity such as raising the minimum wage to a living wage (Hornor, 2017). Similarly, Nurius, Prince and Rocha (2015) recognize that social and material inequalities and marginalization create the conditions of daily life for underprivileged youth, comprising stressors and deficits that apply influence contemporaneously and related to life course trajectories. That said, to promote resilience and thriving in society for all, everyone, including those with greater resources, must be proactive in fostering humanitarian, egalitarian values seen in upstream policies that shape downstream resources for the individual and family. As Bishop Desmond Tutu states "My humanity is bound up with yours, for we can only be human together" (National Volunteer Caregiving Network, n.d., p. 1).

To support prevention through protection as it relates to ACEs, we must recognize that development takes place within interlinked bioecological contexts that comprise a range of environments and societal structures. These consist of the differential provision of risk, such as exposure to abuse and hegemonic belief systems that authenticate or disregard the effects of privilege (Osher et al., 2017). Structural and social characteristics of developmentally rich settings encourage development and protect against adversity when they nurture adults' abilities to accommodate and support children. It is also advantageous when adults impart relevant knowledge, model, and co-regulate the growth of social, emotional, and cognitive capabilities of children. Developmentally rich settings can operate as a constructive web through which complex dynamic skills are cultivated in addition to positive adaptation (Osher et al., 2017).

To have broader positive effects, Turner (2009) states that powerful macro-level influences need to shift from male-controlled, capitalistic, and hegemonic worldview and policies to more gender-neutral, egalitarian, and relational-cultural principles. Furthermore, resources integral to supporting resilience must be distributed more equitably and make certain that the needs of at-risk children and families are met (Turner, 2009). For primary prevention, it must be determined if children really require unique consideration and support, and if this is affirmed, adequate financial resources must be allocated and implemented towards enhancing and upholding resilience-promoting environments for children (Osher et al., 2017). This is critical since children and adults experience macrosystem dynamics directly through attitudes, behaviors, actions, and practices that influence how these individuals experience and respond to situations and circuitously through social stigma and contact with settings where opportunities for enhancement and choice are limited or absent (Osher et al., 2017).

Examining how macrosystem level factors sway resilience building is necessary to clearly perceive the links between ecological levels that are continuously exerting forces on how one is supported or neglected. Illustrations of structural and cultural factors are provided.

Structural macrosystem factors institutionalize practices. This is realized in the case of public and private housing policy that furthers housing segregation which, sequentially, influences wealth accrual. Destructive structural macrosystem factors can similarly be shielded by positive factors. Some exemplars include favorable bonds with neighbors, shared mutual value of one's neighborhood, and a feeling of belonging. Furthermore, advantageous microsystem dynamics can extend by positive factors such as developmental relationships with family members, teachers, and peers (Osher et al., 2017). Cultural macrosystem factors involve hegemonic beliefs and mentalities such as victim-blaming methods to comprehending social dilemmas that discount or deemphasize the effects of history, context, and privilege. Poverty and racism, both distinctly and collectively, cause the occurrence of stress and adversity more expected among children and adults who have to deal repeatedly with the effects of economic adversity and prejudice in their day-to-day lives in settings that disregard the ubiquitous effects of racism (Osher et al., 2017). These consequences may be evident instantly through use of racial slurs, or they may be nascent and merely perceptible upon examination, for example when analyzing racial disparities that are the outcome of numerous small and frequently subtle steps (Osher et al., 2017). Consequences of adversity may likewise be indirect, for example through the effects of housing segregation on the disparity of resources accessible for schools according to subsidies provided locally. The presence of racism is institutionalized in macrosystems via policies and cultural forces that support and systemize racial privilege. In spite of this, we have a choice to foster developmentally rich settings, or not. If we act favorably in accordance with inclusive values we should aspire to embody as a nation, then macrosystem factors will work together with microsystem factors to influence the intergenerational transmission of advantage for many more individuals. Lacking this change and with enduring inequality, housing segregation, education and health disparities, financial hardship, and deficient support for families can cause adult and child effects that place both at risk with a cycle that persists (Osher et al., 2017). The authors believe we should not wait. Change needs to be implemented today. As Mahatma Ghandi states, "The future depends on what you do today" (Leaver, 2016, p. 1).

Raising awareness about the benefits of supporting resilience among policymakers and the general public promotes fostering the building blocks for development of human potential

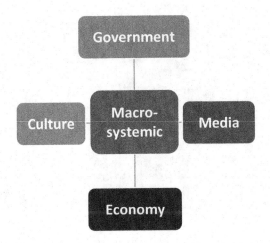

FIGURE 9.2 Examples of Macrosystemic Protective Factors that Promote Resilience

for all using an ecological perspective. Virtuous political systems that support these forms of human rights think of ways to maximize the chances for success and thriving among its people and create an infrastructure and deliver resources to enable its realization in a manner that is acceptable to the people within communities. Broad strategic thinking is required about human potential, approaches to strengthening protective factors, and understanding determinants of resilience (upstream, midstream and downstream) in order to nurture resilience. Moreover, dynamics around structure, strategy, and agency have to be considered when developing prevention through protection initiatives for individuals across the life span (prenatal through adulthood).

In summary, this chapter highlights relevant information about distal systems—exosystem and macrosystem. Importantly we must remember that a dynamic process extends from distal to proximal encompassing ontogenic, microsystem, exosystem (i.e., neighborhood and community settings in which families and children live) and macrosystem. The macrosystem depicts the overarching pattern of the person, micro-and exosystems "characteristic of a given culture or subculture, with particular reference to the belief systems, bodies of knowledge, material resources, customs, lifestyles, opportunity structures, hazards, and life course options that are embedded in each of these broader systems" (Lundberg & Wuermli, 2012, p. 54). Resilience should be nurtured in a multisystemic interactional pattern that is context specific and life course-oriented. Having an ecological appreciation of human development and resilience allows for examination of the influence of community, subculture, and culture on essential psychological and interpersonal practices throughout the life course and (a) the extent these practices facilitate adaptive, positive development and (b) how they may differ with relational, familial, social, and cultural contexts (bidirectional influence between contexts and the individual). Not just a resilient but a thriving civil society necessitates people of character that capture a keener observation of the environments that affect individuals' daily behavior, routines and values. For instance, we know this is necessary for a child because although they are mostly exposed to influences within the micro environment of the family, neither the child nor the family live in a vacuum. Quality of current exo-and-macro

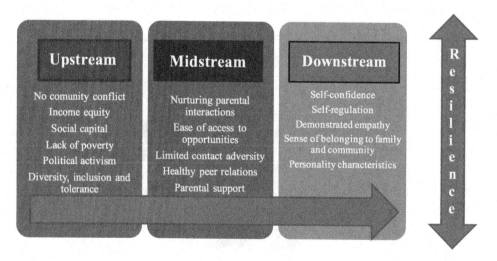

FIGURE 9.3 Distal Systems

environments, including socio-political aspects and individual and family history, impacts one's ability to flourish in life.

Resilience-promoting resources within a multi-level systemic process are not fully effective if systems are not working in concert with each other. All the protective resources should work together to produce a holistic environment. Thus, influence of constantly expanding micro-and macro-level environmental factors establishes a trajectory as to how resilient and thriving children develop into prosocial adolescents and adults.

BOX 9.1 CASE ILLUSTRATION: ELIJAH, 22-YEAR-OLD

Elijah is a 22-year-old African American male admitted to the trauma unit following multiple gunshot wounds to leg, shoulder and abdomen. He is willing to participate in a violence intervention program.

Family history: Single, living in family home with single mother and three siblings. Father is not in the picture. Elijah is currently the support of the family as mother is depressed, uses substances, and is unable to sustain a job. The family is living in poverty in a large east coast city known for its high poverty levels and racial strife. Maternal uncle was killed in the neighborhood 8 years ago in drug-related incident. Elijah has close bond with maternal aunt.

Trauma history: Elijah reports first hearing gunshots in his neighborhood when he was 6 years old. He witnessed his uncle lying on sidewalk after being shot. He lives in a neighborhood with a history of poverty, filled with decaying structures and a known center for drug sales and use in the city.

Adverse childhood experience score: Scoring based on the original study represents (4) ACEs including emotional neglect, mother is a substance abuser, mother has a mental health issue, he was not raised by both biological parents.

Expanded ACE criteria adds (2) ACEs: impact of poverty and impact of community violence.

Health history: Elijah was hospitalized at age 19 following a gunshot wound to his leg; bullet fragments remain. He reports that he was treated in the Emergency Department and released. Both shootings occurred on the street in the process of selling drugs. The first time he was shot, he remembers overhearing nursing staff blaming him for the incident and predicting he would be back in the Emergency Department in the future if he didn't stop selling drugs. He has a history of depression but is not treated. He reports no substance abuse.

Social/emotional composite: Elijah is a quiet but engaging young man who cares about his family. He has a caretaker role with his siblings who look to him as a role model/leader. He reports he is depressed, has difficulty sleeping and reports he has intrusive memories of the shooting during which he thought he would be killed. He is afraid he will have lasting health and mobility problems due to the multiple gunshot wounds. He does not know who will support his family if he does not provide the income. He has been questioned by the police and is concerned about legal ramifications.

Educational/vocational status: Elijah liked school and reports doing well but he left school at age 16 in order to support the family. He later obtained a Graduate Equivalency

Diploma. He has no vocational training. He aspires to go to college and has had an interest in the health professions.

Case: Elijah participated in a violence intervention program in which he was able to obtain financial supports for himself and his family. He healed from his gunshot wounds although he continues to experience abdominal pain and struggles to refrain from use of pain medication. Elijah was supported as he navigated the medical system that was not consistently responsive to his health care needs. He no longer sells drugs. Multiple systems were engaged to assist Elijah. He received counseling for his post-traumatic stress symptoms and was prescribed medication for his depression.

He developed a close relationship with a social worker in the program and participated in support groups, eventually developing a leadership role and mentoring newcomers to the program. Elijah was accepted at his local community college with some financial support. He also obtained a student loan. He completed peer specialist training funded by the city and was hired as a part-time peer specialist. He has stopped attending school in order to focus on his job, with the goal of being hired full-time. Elijah continues to live at home and to use his income to help support his family. He would like to continue his education with the hope of becoming a registered nurse but he cannot continue until he pays back his loan and obtains another loan to fund his further schooling.

Discussion questions:

- What are some of the protective factors—individual, family and community that—contributed to Elijah's resilience?
- What are some of the social determinants of health present in this case?
- What do you think of the various responses of health care professionals to this young man? Do you see yourself in the blaming role when faced with a person whose life circumstances contribute to their injuries?
- What ecosystem elements (context; culture) do you identify in this case?
- How do you think this young man's relatively high Adverse Childhood Experiences score impacts his life?
- Do you see evidence of historical trauma and structural violence in his story?
- What challenges and opportunities are present for Elijah?
- How might the health care and educational systems further support him to achieve his goals?

PART IV

ACE intervention:
A social-ecological approach

10

EARLY IDENTIFICATION AND TRAUMA-INFORMED APPROACHES

Trauma-informed, trauma-responsive, and trauma-sensitive approaches are phrases used largely to communicate actions by human service organizations that strive to preclude and treat the effect of trauma and toxic stress as well as to support and foster resilience. The precise actions linked with trauma-informed methods differ significantly with the service area (e.g. health, mental health, child welfare) and the level of intervention (e.g. prevention, early intervention, treatment) along with the population served (e.g. age cohort, gender, and nature of trauma experience) (Snyder & Lyon, 2017). Currently, the outcomes are disparate in the particular practices with steps toward moving to be a trauma-informed organization.

Nearly two decades ago in North America, psychologists Maxine Harris and Roger Fallot coined the term trauma-informed (Fallot & Harris, 2001). Trauma-informed suggests being sensitive to the traumatic experiences of individuals (e.g., children and parents), families, and entire groups (e.g., Native Americans, African-Americans, lesbian, gay, bisexual, and/ or transgendered individuals) and becoming sensitive to the ways in which trauma impacts organizations and entire systems (criminal justice, courts, and schools). This information allows for a more integrated and appropriate approach to meeting their needs. While trauma-informed care started in organizations that principally serve children and families with considerable histories of trauma for example mental health, juvenile justice, and child welfare systems, the desire is to employ the principles of trauma-informed care so that we can support youth to heal from traumatic experiences which are pervasive in our society (Snyder & Lyon, 2017). Ordinarily, maternal and child health programs are implicated in delivering primary care and prevention services for children and families. Prevention and early intervention produces an opportunity to employ trauma-informed principles in a setting that underscores protective factors and resilience in addition to healing (Snyder & Lyon, 2017).

Kaufman (2017) further described that to be trauma-informed indicates that one is:

> educated about the impact of interpersonal violence and victimization on an individual's life and development ... Trauma-informed practice recognizes the ways in which trauma impacts systems and individuals. Becoming trauma-informed which can be considered a primary level intervention results in the recognition that behavioral symptoms, mental

health diagnosis, and involvement in the criminal justice system are all manifestations of injury, rather than indicators of sickness or badness—the two current explanations for such behavior.

(p. 1220)

A trauma-informed approach can take place in practically any setting including communities. Utilizing this approach does not compel disclosure of trauma. However, the setting must be cognizant about what is known in relation to trauma, as well as its prevalence, its extensive and profound effect on survivors, and the multifaceted and varied ways that individuals recover and heal from trauma. Also, it is important to understand that re-traumatizing clientele or families can occur based on how the health professional or organization offers services and interacts with these individuals. Sensitivity to the person's experiences and needs is critical to their development and wellbeing; therefore relating in a trauma-informed way *does no harm* and efforts are made to treat each other as valuable human beings. These perspectives are aligned with assumptions set forth by the Substance Abuse and Mental Health Services Administration's (SAMHSAs) concept of trauma-informed as it relates to a program, organization, or system indicating the importance of:

1. Realizing the pervasive effect of trauma and conceivable paths for recovery;
2. Recognizing the signs and symptoms of trauma among those affected (e.g., clients, families, staff, and others embroiled with the system);
3. Responding "by integrating knowledge about trauma into policies, procedures, and practices" (p. 387);
4. Resisting the potential to re-traumatize an individual

(Bloom, 2016)

Six key principles that SAMHSA upholds as essential for a trauma-informed approach include: (a) safety, (b) trustworthiness and transparency, (c) peer support, (d) collaboration and mutuality, (e) empowerment, voice and choice, and (f) cultural, historical, and gender issues (SAMHSA: Project Aware, 2014). The practices based in the guiding principles and understanding of trauma allow workers to provide services that are more supportive and less retraumatizing compared to services that lack an understanding of trauma and its impacts. A crucial aspect of trauma-informed methods is that it is an extremely tailored process to the individual that includes continuous reflection and work. This paradigm or cultural shift relates that trauma-informed practices are to an extent a "way of being" rather than about adhering to a pre-specified procedure or clinical intervention for how each person is engaged. More specifically, trauma-informed practices implement universal precautions with each person an organization makes contact with. This is an intentional process of change, with multiple-level strategies including detecting obstacles; employing systems and processes throughout the entire organization; attending to employee wellness and safety; and affording education skills and support for employees to support their success with the approach.

As we engage individuals with histories of trauma a paradigm shift is required. Words used carry power and meaning; therefore we should cease asking, "What's wrong with you?" or approach clients thinking "How can I fix you" and instead ask, "What has happened to you (Bloom, 2016, p. 385)?" And "What do you need to support your development and recovery (DeCandia & Guarino, 2015)?" There are some challenges with implementing trauma-informed approaches such as:

TABLE 10.1 Explanation of SAMSHA Trauma-Informed Principles (SAMHSA: Project Aware, 2014)

Principle	Description	Examples of Operationalizing the Principle
Safety	• Organizational staff and individuals served at all ages feel physically and psychologically safe. • Interpersonal relations foster feelings of safety. • Appreciating safety as described by individuals served.	• Ask approval for a professional student's engagement during a physical with your health care practitioner.
Trustworthiness and Transparency	• Organizational processes and decisions are made with transparency. The aim is to develop and preserve trust with individuals and family members as well as with staff, and others having something to do with the organization.	• Clearly lay out processes for promotion within an organization.
Peer Support	• Recovery is important and much support is received by other persons with lived experiences of trauma (i.e., trauma survivors). For persons who are quite young this individual may be family members who experienced trauma.	• Employee recruitment must strive to capture candidates with diverse lived experiences including trauma survivors.
Collaboration and Mutuality	• Healing from trauma occurs through meaningful relationships. • Within these relationships, it is essential to level power distinctions among all staff regardless of role. • All organization personnel engage in a trauma-informed manner implementing therapeutic practices.	• Partner with the client in determining which goals on the treatment plan will the primary focus for the visit.
Empowerment, Voice, and Choice	• Strengths of individuals are acknowledged, appreciated, and nurtured including recognizing that individuals, organizations, and communities can heal. • Development of additional skills is acquired as needed.	• Allow client to share their ideas regarding best approaches to attain a healthy weight and offer several alternatives that they may also consider.
Cultural, Historical, and Gender Issues	• Organizations encompass policies, practices, and procedures deemed to be responsive to cultural, racial, and ethnic needs of their clientele in a manner that is gender-responsive. • Appreciating and understanding historical trauma is realized and is considered in the development of the aforementioned points.	• Be attentive to both covert and overt biases realizing that your life experience is not that of others given dissimilarities in life opportunity.

a   Limited empirical research on implementation science of trauma-informed approaches as well as how to best direct resources to capitalize on the greatest impact;

b   Requiring a shift in language and a need to develop best practices encompassing this subject area, with some promoting a stronger focus on toxic stress and/or resiliency;

c   Having to lead efforts beyond ACEs training and shifting emphasis to supplying staff with tools required to effectively meet the demands of individuals who have experienced trauma and delivering training on how to apply trauma-informed approaches;

d   Necessitating organizational time and expense needed to assess all of the policies and practices within the organization in addition to transforming them into trauma-informed models;

e   Needing to have strong leaders championing for and driving persistent organizational change (Clervil & DeCandia, 2013; Loveland, 2017); and finally

f   Requiring an understanding that the organization is a living system that requires change which inherently involves risk (Bloom, 2017).

These barriers do not outweigh the benefits. The benefits of trauma-informed methods support fostering well-being for individuals and health organizations, better teamwork, greater work satisfaction, and less injuries (Bloom, 2017). Importantly, it does not solve past trauma; however it presents consistency and clarity with survivors understanding the practice of staff with their professional roles and demonstrates humanness. Also, by improved understanding of ACEs and trauma a common language and framework is cultivated to better recognize and take action in an effective and compassionate manner on behavioral problems confronted in many organizations (Loveland, 2017). As Bloom (2017) states, "a mission driven, trauma-responsive organization is an organization that counteracts the short-term and long-term effects of stress, adversity and trauma on its managers, staff, and the people it serves while staying true to its mission, expanding social justice and improving the health and well-being of all organizational stakeholders" (p. 11). Additional benefits are located in Figure 10.1.

As noted by San Francisco's Trauma Informed Systems Initiative (2014), Bloom imparted that to be really trauma-informed the system must develop and continuously nurture a process of understanding itself. Likewise, a program can only be safe for clientele if it is

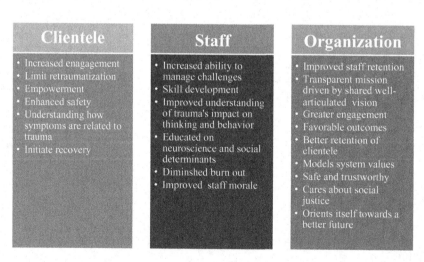

FIGURE 10.1 Benefits of Utilizing Trauma-Informed Principles (Bloom, 2016; Gilliver, 2016)

concurrently safe for both staff and administrators. Absent such a process and regardless of well-intentioned training endeavors, no real system transformation will happen. Actually, many systems for the most part are trauma-organized where repeating of undesirable behaviors occur, instead of healing the wounds formerly experienced by clientele and staff (San Francisco's Trauma Informed Systems Initiative, 2014).

Quite importantly, we must also understand that even in the most forward thinking, well-considered trauma-informed models there is a risk of covering up the status quo (Becker-Blease, 2017). When that takes place, there is danger of criticizing those who have been wounded for not seizing the benefits of or welcoming the progressive services. Moreover, there is danger of dishonoring, silencing, and retraumatizing those wounded, telling them that their needs are met, when in effect this could be furthest from reality (Becker-Blease, 2017). Speaking about the value of trauma-informed care only will not work. Meaningful action is needed that is aligned with spoken trauma-informed values: for example, decreasing implicit and explicit bias among members of hiring committees along with (a) policies concerning how candidates are interviewed, (b) identifying whose responsibility it is to oversee institutional behaviors and the organizational climate, and personal reflection and education about one's own implicit and explicit biases, and (c) monitoring how power differences get in the way of achieving optimal organizational functioning (Becker-Blease, 2017).

A secondary level of intervention is trauma responsiveness, which is essentially "walking the talk" by putting into practice what we know and moving beyond being trauma-informed. Thus, a change in behavior in addition to gaining knowledge is requisite. A trauma-responsive workplace promotes an atmosphere that increases empowerment for staffs at all levels (Handran, 2013). Consequently, everyone is not only educated to ensure that they were trauma-informed, but a workplace would additionally create particular practices and policies within the organization to prevent trauma. Moreover, a trauma-responsive environment would intentionally attempt to diminish the risk of causing things to be harmful for individuals or families who have experienced trauma and capitalize on improvement (Handran, 2013). In addition, staff within these workplaces are emboldened to take part in self-care activities consisting of nutritional (e.g., eating right), psychological (e.g., mindfulness techniques), physical (e.g., fitness routines), emotional (e.g., socializing with others whose companionship one enjoys), spiritual (e.g., prayer or connection with nature), and balance (e.g., work-home-play/rest balance) (Handran, 2013). Importantly, a trauma-responsive environment would similarly establish a dense system of networks with community resources that could deliver trauma-specific treatment (Handran, 2013).

Organizationally, when a traumatic event occurs its reactions are frequently analogous to the individual's responses. Bloom (2017) argues that organizations, akin to individuals, are "living, complex, adaptive systems and that being alive, they are vulnerable to stress, particularly chronic and repetitive stress" (p. 6). The precedence of a trauma-informed system is to encourage openness, however frequently stress is managed by enhanced rigidity. This condition results in tension spreading throughout the workplace; notably, our traditional approach to these circumstances and correspondingly human nature is to generate added rules and regulations to thwart more problems. These automatic reactions may in fact detract from quality of care and result in staff and clients feeling confounded (Handran, 2013). Organizational and individual standards of practice must be in place to provide the best care to traumatized populations to safeguard clients and promote efforts with delivering superior services; as well, staff must be supported by mitigating burnout and diminishing the potential for vicarious trauma. Essentially, trauma-responsive organizational cultures incite trauma awareness, prevention, and acceptance; in addition, organizations must confirm and understand the effect of vicarious trauma. When organizations lack insight about vicarious trauma they are at greater risk of becoming burnt out or trauma-organized (Handran, 2013).

A tertiary intervention for ACEs is trauma-specific (e.g., trauma-centered or trauma-focused) since the emphasis is on the sequelae of trauma and facilitating recovery. Thus, clinical interventions are the focus of trauma-specific services, while trauma-informed care focuses on organizational culture and practice (DeCandia, Guarino, & Clervil, 2014). Bloom (2015) states that trauma-focused strategies are about including in the discussion and processing of the traumatic event throughout the treatment, typically as stand-alone, manualized procedures. Trauma-centered however is represented by an intermediate approach; as such, the examination of the trauma is carried out during the early stages of therapy and then is employed as an underpinning as the therapy shifts into present issues. SAMHSA: Project Aware (2014) suggests that trauma-specific approaches represent evidence-based and promising prevention, intervention, or treatment services that attend to traumatic stress along with any co-occurring disorders that surfaced during or after trauma. It is important for trauma-informed organizations to embrace trauma-specific interventions that operate along with screening for trauma. Some specific examples of trauma-specific interventions include eye movement desensitization reprocessing (EMDR), cognitive processing therapy, prolonged exposure (PE), trauma-focused cognitive behavior therapy, and crisis intervention stress debriefing (CISD). Many of the treatments for trauma indicated as evidence based or promising have treated Post-Traumatic Stress Disorder. Notably, trauma-specific care must consider cultural factors since they contribute to the various forms of trauma a person may experience as well as the risk for ongoing trauma. Moreover, consideration must be given to how individuals manage and communicate their experiences in addition to taking into account the form of care that would be most effective.

Considering the three areas—trauma-informed (primary)/responsive (secondary)/specific (tertiary) interventions having the detailed information shared above enables us to clearly speak to resources needed for effecting positive change to tackle these problems. Given the evolving effort to improve recovery and build resilience for trauma survivors, an array of treatments should be offered (e.g., mind/body, trauma-focused cognitive behavioral therapy, experiential approaches and expressive therapies, including: mindfulness programs, trauma-sensitive yoga, and expressive art therapies such as psychodrama), emphasizing both verbal and inclusion of non-verbal approaches that aid in the therapeutic relationship and the formation of safety and trust (Buck, Bean, & de Marco, 2017). Considering this, further deliberation is needed to determine what modifications are needed in research as well as policy measures (Bloom, 2016). Policy is burdened with compromise, and while trauma-informed programs may not completely realize all principles of trauma-informed care continually, it is doubtful that any particular policy or legislation article would completely manifest all the principles either (Bowen & Murshid, 2016). Trauma-informed principles laid out by SAMHSA offer a conceptual model whose policies in action may manifest to differing degrees (Bowen & Murshid, 2016). A commonality through all the trauma-informed principles is that their sanctioning infers a significant amount of consideration and resources upstream as it relates to social determinants of health (Bowen & Murshid, 2016). Even though there is an expense attributed to numerous upstream policy activities, it is likely that substantial economic savings will occur along with the prevention of human suffering given that trauma would prevent or mitigate its primary health effects (Bowen & Murshid, 2016). The continuum of descriptions (e.g., trauma-informed [primary], trauma-responsive [secondary], and trauma-specific [tertiary] interventions) supports a way to best evaluate diverse policies centered on the level of intervention a policy is intended to affect (Bloom, 2016). Consequently, a trauma-informed policy could give push for the primary prevention measures; these are often invisible when meaningful discourse occurs at the policy level (Bloom, 2016). Trauma-responsive policies would have an opportunity to be explicitly created to diminish harm and extend opportunities for healthy growth and development among people at risk. Then trauma-specific policymaking would be in a better position to create and maintain effective interventions that alleviate the effects of traumatic experience and foster healing (Bloom, 2016). Health professionals, particularly those who work with trauma-affected populations and communities, must support policy to integrate a trauma-informed focus. This is requisite in order to shape policy to better manifest the realities of lived experience; it is essential that policymakers be informed directly from those confronted with these issues, such as health professionals delivering service and service users, with the aim to educate policymakers regarding the significance of trauma-informed principles and how policies can display them (Bowen & Murshid, 2016). The present-day reality is that even health professionals delivering service at the highest quality of trauma-informed care must obtain their clientele from and discharge them to a society and a social order that are for the most part not trauma-informed (Bowen & Murshid, 2016). Trauma-informed policy advocacy proposes an opportunity for increasingly shifting this reality (Bowen & Murshid, 2016).

In the following sections, we will examine trauma interventions for the individual, family, and schools realizing that nonpathologizing approaches to healing are important (Gómez et al., 2016). As stated by Karen Saakvitne "Everyone has a right to have a future that is not dictated by the past" (Peters & Silvestri, 2016, p. 1).

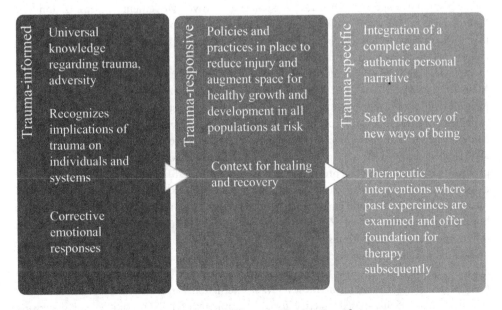

FIGURE 10.2 Continuum: Trauma-Informed Through Trauma-Specific

Individuals, families and groups

While this section will be examining some of the individual, family and group interventions for trauma, it is worthwhile to highlight that as a society, we have an extensive history of alternately refuting and focusing on traumatic stress as the root of suffering (Bloom, 2000; DeCandia & Guarino, 2015). This influences where most of the attention and blame is placed for an individual's wellbeing. When trauma is refuted, the paradigm of both personal responsibility and pathology is the central voice encouraging a "blame the victim" mindset. However, when given high attention using an alternate lens, social context and the effect of environment, experience, and relationships on human development are core components of cause of, and key to, human suffering (DeCandia & Guarino, 2015). We must remove our blinders and be honest about the realism and scale of trauma (e.g., violence and abuse) in our society, including those who are most at risk and why this is the case. There are strong emotions associated with this truth and some may see this as too much to bear (DeCandia & Guarino, 2015); however, the larger society does not have the luxury to remain in denial mode regarding the cost associated with remedying the problem and actually precluding trauma from occurring in the first place (Bloom, 2000). It is important to realize that denial permits us to detach ourselves from the strong emotions and moral duty to act. The effects contribute to pathology and interventions that are located within the individual instead of the broader social sphere (DeCandia & Guarino, 2015). Nevertheless, this chapter will highlight several treatments for trauma for adults and children including eye movement desensitization and reprocessing; prolonged exposure therapy; seeking safety; trauma-focused cognitive behavioral therapy; child-parent psychotherapy; attachment, self-regulation, and competency; trauma recovery and empowerment model; and creative arts therapies. The next chapter will look at larger societal and macro level treatment intervention for trauma.

In 1989, Shapiro developed the *eye movement desensitization and reprocessing* (EMDR) method, which includes a brief exposure to trauma-related images while clients track the therapist's rapid finger movements with their eye. Eye Movement Desensitization and Reprocessing, a structured and integrated psychotherapy combining different well-established psychotherapeutic techniques (such as imagined exposure, resource development, cognitive change, and self-control) with bilateral sensory stimulation, is an information processing therapy for treatment of emotionally distressing traumatic events (Chen et al., 2018; Menschner & Maul, 2016; Pagani et al., 2018). EMDR is based on the adaptive information processing model, according to which a high level of disturbance caused by traumatic experiences results in a failure of the information processing system to properly elaborate and contextualize into the semantic memory network the autobiographical event (Pagani et al., 2018). Specifically, it is an 8-phase program: (1) history and treatment planning; (2) preparation; (3) assessment; (4) reprocessing and desensitization; (5) installation; (6) body scan; (7) closure; (8) re-evaluation of past, present, and future. EMDR relies upon stressful recollections coupled with the use of alternating bilateral tactile or auditory stimulation as well as brief eye movement sets of ~30 to achieve its goals. Through EMDR the dysfunctional stored experiences will be transformed into adaptive ones, consolidating them into the natural neural processes of memory (Pagani et al., 2018). Importantly, EMDR does not require intensive prolonged exposure to the traumatic experiences (Chen et al., 2018). Recently EMDR has been included in the most relevant international trauma treatment guidelines and considered as evidence-based practice for the treatment of PTSD, anxiety and depression symptoms (Pagani et al., 2018). Its target population includes adults who have experienced trauma or who have been diagnosed with PTSD. The clinical impact of EMDR has been proven by several investigations also demonstrating a clear association between symptoms disappearance and changes in cortical structure and functionality (Laugharne et al., 2016; Pagani et al., 2018). It is endorsed by the World Health Organization and Department of Veterans Affairs (Menschner & Maul, 2016).

Prolonged exposure therapy, developed by psychologist Edna Foa for adult populations, is an efficacious and effective evidence-based treatment for Post-Traumatic Stress Disorder (PTSD) and related problems (McLean, Yeh, Rosenfield, & Foa, 2015). Prolonged exposure therapy, a cognitive behavioral therapy method intended to aid sufferers to emotionally process their traumatic experience, comprises varied strategies including repeated recounting of the trauma and exposure to dreaded real-life circumstances. It also consists of breathing techniques to reduce the physiological experience of stress and talking through the trauma (Menschner & Maul, 2016). Prolonged exposure therapy is a derivative of emotional processing theory, which highlights the role of harmful trauma-related cognitions the person holds about themselves such as "I'm incompetent" or holds about the world including the world is completely unsafe, nobody can be trusted," promoting the development and maintenance of PTSD (McLean et al., 2015). Recovery ensues when erroneous, undesirable trauma-related cognitions are refuted through thinking and speaking about the trauma and/or managing trauma reminders in everyday life. Recovery also develops by grasping that thinking and tackling trauma cues do not cause the expected harm (McLean et al., 2015). In prolonged exposure therapy, alteration of these cognitions is accomplished by assisting clients to deal with trauma-related stimuli and conditions (in-vivo exposure); next reexamining and processing the traumatic memory (imaginal exposure) lacking the threat is required (Blankenship, 2017; McLean et al., 2015). This treatment usually consists of eight to 15, 60 to 90-minute sessions that happen one to two times weekly. Prolonged exposure therapy is recognized as the most empirically adopted treatment for PTSD; of 25 randomized control trials, prolonged exposure therapy demonstrated favorable outcomes for diminishing PTSD symptoms, effectively for both acute and chronic PTSD (Blankenship, 2017). Positive improvements have been sustained for at least one year and this treatment has been adopted by the Veterans Heath Administration, leading to a national initiative to properly educate their clinicians in prolonged exposure therapy (Blankenship, 2017).

Seeking Safety, developed by Lisa Najavitis, is unique in that it is one of the most broadly used integrated programs for concurrent treatment of substance abuse and trauma (Najavits, 2002). Also, this model was initially established as an empowerment model for women; however it is presently known as being an effective and extensively used method for others such as traumatized United States veterans. Seeking Safety is therefore beneficial for both men and women who have experienced trauma, or who have been diagnosed with PTSD or substance use issues and is utilized in correctional facilities, mental health centers and residential treatment centers (Giordano et al., 2016). The Seeking Safety Model is an evidence-based, present-focused program established principally on cognitive-behavioral techniques to assist individuals to achieve safety from both trauma/PTSD and substance abuse. Seeking safety is founded on five fundamental concepts: (a) safety as the priority for treatment; (b) integration of PTSD and substance use treatment; (c) a focus on ideals; (d) content focused on cognitive, behavioral, interpersonal and case management; and (e) attention to clinician processes (Menschner & Maul, 2016). Treatment is adaptable and employs 25 different areas that examine both cognitive and behavioral areas, such as coping with triggers, regaining control over substances and setting boundaries in relationships, and is suitable for both group and individual counseling structures (Najavits, 2002). Regarding outcomes for this model, Menschner and Maul (2016) record Seeking Safety as supported by research evidence specifically for adults by the California Evidence-Based Clearinghouse and it is indicated as having strong research support for adults by the Society of Addiction Psychology of the American Psychological Association.

Trauma-focused cognitive behavioral therapy, developed by Judith Cohen, Anthony Mannarino, and Esther Deblinger as a psychosocial treatment modality, integrates trauma-sensitive interventions, cognitive-behavioral principles, along with facets of attachment, developmental neurobiology, family, empowerment, and humanistic theoretical models with the aim of optimally attending to the needs of traumatized children and families (Blankenship, 2017). Trauma-focused cognitive behavioral therapy places emphasis on three key areas, including tackling distorted beliefs and ascriptions linked to abuse or trauma; affording a caring environment for children to reveal traumatic experiences; and assisting parents who are not abusive to manage their own distress and acquire skills to support their children (Menschner & Maul, 2016; Racco & Vis, 2015). This type of therapy is meant to decrease negative emotions and behaviors associated with child sexual abuse, domestic violence, and trauma (Menschner & Maul, 2016). The typical number of sessions employing trauma-focused cognitive behavioral therapy in treating PTSD is 12 to 18 among youth, ages 3–21, and parents or caregivers who have experienced abuse or trauma (Blankenship, 2017; Racco & Vis, 2015). According to Menschner and Maul (2016) trauma-focused cognitive behavioral therapy has been underscored by the National Child Traumatic Stress Network, the California Evidence-based Clearinghouse, and SAMHSA as a model program or promising treatment practice.

Child-parent psychotherapy is an evidence-based, manualized treatment focused on children aged birth to 5 years who have experienced traumatic stress and, consequently, are experiencing behavioral concerns, attachment problems, and/or signs of early mental health problems (Perry & Conners-Burrow, 2016). The central goal of child-parent psychotherapy is to bolster the caregiver-child relationship to rebuild the child's feeling of safety and attachment and to enhance the child's outcomes (Menschner & Maul, 2016). Essential aspects of child-parent psychotherapy comprise psychoeducation about trauma as well as child development, enhancing safety, behavioral management, affective regulation, processing of the trauma, improving the child-parent relationship, and continuity of daily living (Perry & Conners-Burrow, 2016). Child-parent psychotherapy is characteristically provided in weekly sessions during a span of one year. Child-parent psychotherapy is supported by the National Registry of Evidence-Based Programs and Practices as well as by research evidence from the California Evidence-Based Clearinghouse for Child Welfare (Menschner & Maul, 2016; Perry & Conners-Burrow, 2016).

Attachment, self-regulation, and competency is a framework based in theory and empirical knowledge regarding the effects of trauma, recognizing the core effects of trauma exposure on self-regulation, attachment, and developmental competencies, which calls attention to the significance of understanding and intervening with the child-in-context (Kinniburgh, Blaustein, Spinazzola, & van der Kolk, 2005). Also, this framework both (a) rests on the belief that systemic change contributes to effective and sustainable outcomes and (b) functions as a guide to choose treatment options, while acknowledging the need for individually tailored interventions along with the critical role of each practitioner's skill base (Kinniburgh et al., 2005).

The aim of the attachment, self-regulation, and competency approach is to attend to vulnerabilities produced by exposure to devastating life conditions that hamper healthy development. Through developing skills, alleviating internal torment, and bolstering the security of the caregiving system, interventions directed by this framework endeavor to afford children generalizable tools that improve resilient outcome. The attachment, self-regulation, and competency approach focuses on youth aged 2–21 years, as well as families who have experienced chronic traumatic stress, multiple traumas, and/or continuing exposure to adverse life experiences. Menschner and Maul (2016) submit that outcomes from the attachment, self-regulation, and competency approach generates a diminution in a child's post-traumatic stress symptoms and overall mental health symptoms, along with increased adaptive and social skills.

Trauma, Recovery and Empowerment Model, developed by Fallot and Harris in the early 1990s, is fully manualized and was originally created as a gender-specific group intervention to help female survivors of trauma who also have substance use issues and/or serious mental illness. Pulling from cognitive restructuring, skills-training techniques and psychoeducation, the 18 to 29 session intervention stresses the development of both coping skills and social support including topics associated with empowerment, trauma education, and skill-building (Fallot & Harris, 2002). While the Trauma, Recovery and Empowerment Model was initially developed entirely for women, adaption has been made in order to meet the complex needs of male trauma-survivors (Fallot & Harris, 2001). Giordano and colleagues (2016) state the trauma, recovery and empowerment model has demonstrated efficacy in various settings including community mental health agencies and residential substance abuse treatment centers.

Creative arts approaches (i.e., music, art, dance/movement, and drama therapy), used to treat trauma since the 1970s, are right-brain dominant and may permit trauma to be retrieved through sensory processes. With these practices, treatment of trauma is established on the belief that the verbal portion of the brain shuts down as a result of traumatic experiences and consequently the memory of the trauma is stowed covertly through bodily sensations instead of overtly through language and cognitions (Dauber, Lotsos, & Pulido, 2015). Therefore, the exclusive use of talk therapy with traumatized individuals (across the lifespan) may not enable entrée to the trauma memory, which is kept in the non-verbal portion of the brain. Integration of creative ways of expression supports expression of these unspoken memories in a nonverbal way, thus setting the foundation for later integration of the trauma narrative (Dauber et al., 2015). The evidence, however, informing their efficacy lacks systematic assessment. Nevertheless, Baker and colleagues (Baker, Metcalf, Varker, & O'Donnell, 2017) have suggested these processes by which creative art therapies may well improve PTSD symptoms:

a   Relaxation experienced during creative art therapy could reduce hyperarousal.
b   Nonverbal expression facilitates the expression of memories and emotions that are difficult to put into words, as both art and trauma are sensory mediated.
c   Containment of traumatic material within a creative art product provides a sense of control, empowerment, agency, and accomplishment.
d   Symbolic expression makes progressive exposure tolerable and helps overcome avoidance.

e   The pleasure of creation builds self-esteem, helps rekindle responsiveness to rewards, and reduces emotional numbness.

f   The activation of emotional behavior and sensory emotional processing through creative engagement leads to stress and directly affects the areas of the brain that are associated with post-traumatic expressions.

(Baker et al., 2017, p. 2)

These are only a snapshot of selective treatments with varying levels of evidence associated with them for individual, parent-child, or group-level trauma treatment interventions. Before any type of treatment is recommended, the licensed health professional partners with the client to choose a therapy modality that best corresponds to their client population and mutually agreed upon goals. As knowledge concerning the nature of post-traumatic responses has progressed over time, there is a broader awareness for the fact that trauma responses are normal reactions to aberrant situations (Buck et al., 2017). There needs to be ongoing evaluations of current and new modalities underway. Health professionals must have access to an extended collection of treatment selections that consist of modalities intended to explicitly attend to the embodiment of trauma, particularly given that the great majority of mental and behavioral therapies are talk-based. We know that along with the influences that trauma has on the brain, trauma likewise lives in the muscles, bones, and the neurons operating in the musculoskeletal system (Buck et al., 2017). Similarly, when the limbic system is frequently activated during stress responses, there is a heightened risk that it will persist and place the body in a hypervigilant condition. Obviously, traditional psychotherapy experiences can feel unsafe to clients especially with their systems being already overwhelmed. Also, talk-based therapy alone tends to be declared ineffective especially when the consequences of trauma on the body are blended with the outcomes of trauma on cognitive processes. This is particularly true for individuals who endured their first traumatic experiences as children (Buck et al., 2017). Moreover, attaining quality and effective interventions with adequate access allows for diminished intergeneration transmission of ACEs. Through individual, familial and group interventions as well as proactive steps with universal education, strategies for trauma-informed parenting can be cultivated to avoid the intergenerational transmission of ACEs. Specifically, Family and Children Services (2018) argue that three core protective systems that assist children and adults surmount the effects and intergenerational transfer of ACEs: 1) strengthen individual competencies and skills in people; 2) enhance the attachment that youth have with caring, competent, and empathetic individuals especially those who they have frequent contact; and 3) foster a protective community that nurtures empowerment.

Schools

"Trauma-informed schools can heal children out of trauma rather than discipline them because of it."
Barbara Oehlberg (Capatosto, 2015, p. 1)

It is rare that a child who crosses the doorway of a school does not transport with them a reservoir of trauma (Paccione-Dyszlewski, 2016). Whether this hurt and anguish from trauma is the size of a pencil case, backpack, or large piece of luggage, the chances are that some level of trauma exists and it is painful (Paccione-Dyszlewski, 2016). As we have highlighted in earlier chapters, children who experience trauma have an increased probability of acquiring a variety of physical, mental/emotional health, and behavioral difficulties (Anderson, Blitz, & Saastamoinen, 2015). What's more, we know that, living in poverty as well as experiencing loss, abuse, and violence produces neurophysiological stress responses that likely interfere with a child's ability to independently regulate their emotions and behavior (Anderson et al., 2015). Quite often, these are the children branded as "difficult students" attributable to their challenging behaviors. These children are also frequently transferred to alternative programs, which functions as a pipeline to prison (Anderson et al., 2015). Integrating trauma-informed approaches in a strategic and comprehensive manner in school communities is vital to effectively meet the multifaceted needs of children who encounter astounding adversity (Anderson et al., 2015). Moreover, the endorsement of trauma-informed education is championed by the National Education Association, which acknowledges the importance of trauma-informed practices and preferably approaching students' behaviors from a more constructive manner (Phifer & Hall, 2016). The trauma-informed movement in schools has been led by a select few including Susan Cole with the Massachusetts Advocates for Children and the Trauma and Learning Policy Initiative, Ron Hertel with the Compassionate Schools Initiative in Washington State, Jennifer Sanders with the Ohio Department of Youth Services, and Nic Dibble with the Wisconsin Department of Public Instruction (Phifer & Hall, 2016).

Importantly, childhood symptomology and later-life effects of student trauma have an enormous influence on the educational system. Consequently, schools must not only provide quality instruction on reading, writing, and thinking; they have to concentrate equally on growing into an epicenter of social and emotional development (Paccione-Dyszlewski, 2016). Fortuitously, educational practices that are conscious of this effect can produce a meaningful shift in how schools identify and apply prevention and healing processes. A fundamental conception of a trauma-informed venue is that everybody who interacts with a student presumes that each child has trauma as part of his/her background and behaves accordingly (Anderson et al., 2015). Consequently, educators must understand the symptoms of toxic stress and trauma as well as how these experiences present within the school setting. The climate set by educators can produce a caring, gentler environment where children feel uninhibited to divulge their trauma. A culture grounded in trust and acceptance is valuable and incredibly positive toward forming a constructive learning atmosphere that also can heal and transcend the effects of toxic stress (Paccione-Dyszlewski, 2016). Yaroshefsky and Shwedel (2015) argue that it is of the essence that any trauma-informed care program in schools be employed to all children and not concentrate exclusively on children classified with trauma exposure. There is an association between success for all students when there is cohesion in teaching spaces where trauma-informed care approaches were adopted for the whole school. This approach creates less conflict and disorganization; accordingly, the trauma-informed approach is advantageous for all children in the school, not simply those who have been exposed to traumatic experiences (Yaroshefsky & Shwedel, 2015). A move in school culture to transition to be more trauma-informed will allow maximum academic growth. Otherwise, by not recognizing and taking appropriate responses to mitigate damaging childhood experiences, the toxicity of trauma will destroy the very potential of learning (Paccione-Dyszlewski, 2016).

Integration of trauma-informed principles in educational contexts necessitates that both students and staff develop knowledge about trauma and its effects. This understanding influences the services supplied to the student, which are presented within a trusting relationship between educators and youth which has the ability to heal students from trauma and prevent concurrent trauma from occurring (Fallot & Harris, 2001); the authors of this paper see this as a true paradigm shift from experiences normally provided in educational settings especially for

Similarly, Chafouleas, Johnson, Overstreet, and Santos (2016) speak about another trauma-informed service delivery model for the school—the School Wide Positive Behavior Interventions and Supports. This program accentuates that the essential elements of capacity building needed to attain effective, school-wide implementation of trauma-informed practice consists of training, coaching, and behavioral expertise. These elements are quite important for trauma-informed service delivery models since the majority of educators and school-based mental health professionals lack training in trauma or trauma-informed approaches (Chafouleas et al., 2016). An educational workforce must be (a) knowledgeable about vicarious traumatization and trauma including its effects on development, (b) able to utilize skills and strategies that avert and reduce its effect on children, (c) adept at de-escalation strategies to prevent re-traumatization of students, (d) informed about meaningful self-care techniques; this is sometimes referred to as obtaining Trauma 101 training. Lacking this type of knowledge and training, school personnel will likely not recognize or understand the link between a child's presentation, behaviors, and symptoms and exposure to trauma (Chafouleas et al., 2016). Take for example school personnel who misinterpret trauma-related behaviors as oppositional or defiant behavior, mistakenly using harsh punishment approaches that can function as triggers for students who have been traumatized. This also allows for failed opportunities to support social, emotional, and academic growth. This form of training in trauma and trauma-informed care is aimed at building the knowledge, skills, and motivation needed for the implementation of trauma-informed approaches (Chafouleas et al., 2016).

While essential, this form of training alone is not enough to ensure effective and efficient application of trauma-informed approaches. This training must be supplemented and strengthened through more concentrated trainings that place emphasis on specific trauma-informed classroom approaches and by coaching teachers to enhance their capacity to employ trauma-informed skills and strategies (Chafouleas et al., 2016). Professional development and coaching for teachers creates individual-level competencies in trauma-informed care. This must be further enhanced with organizational competencies and supporting infrastructure for school-wide trauma-informed practices to be embraced and applied effectively (Chafouleas et al., 2016). Finally, leadership within the school may also need technical support to deliver the structure and tools for school-wide operationalization such as thinking and planning as well as engagement in data-based decision-making for the systemic implementation and monitoring of trauma-informed approaches (Chafouleas et al., 2016).

Health care professionals who function in school settings are uniquely situated at the crosswalk of health and education in settings which support reduction in obstacles including cost and transportation. Such settings also allow health professionals to respond to childhood adversity, enhance prevention and early intervention efforts given the opportunity for coordinated physical and mental health services. At the crux of school-based health centers embedded in a school or collaborative link of a school with another entity providing services (e.g., health system partnerships such as hospitals, federally qualified health care centers and look alikes as well as health departments), is the partnership between the schools and health organizations that offer support and services to the students (School-Based Health Alliance, 2017). Schools perform a vital role in the health of youth and healthy children are more prone to attend school ready to learn. School-based health centers provide comprehensive health services in schools where students often have trust, familiarity and accessibility to services therefore they may almost be a one-stop site for primary care, mental health, oral health and health prevention services. For a matter of fact some have such comprehensive services

TABLE 10.2 Resource Table: Examples of Additional Trauma-Informed Schools

Trauma-Informed Model	Resource Link
Trauma-Sensitive Schools	http://traumasensitiveschools.org/tlpi-publications/download-a-free-copy-of-a-guide-to-creating-trauma-sensitive-schools/
The Trauma-Informed School: A Step-by-Step Implementation Guide for Administrators and School Personnel	http://www.beyondconsequences.com/the-trauma-informed-school
Healthy Environments and Response to Trauma in Schools	http://coe.ucsf.edu/coe/spotlight/ucsf_hearts.html
Multiplying Connections	http://www.multiplyingconnections.org/become-trauma-informed/tools-become-trauma-informed
Making SPACE for Learning	http://det.wa.edu.au/childprotection/detcms/inclusiveeducation/child-protection/public/files/making-space-for-learning—trauma-informed-practice-in-schools.en
Compassionate Schools Project	http://www.k12.wa.us/CompassionateSchools/

they can serve as medical homes for students along with coordinating health care services by numerous providers who assist in managing chronic conditions. Data from the School-Based Health Alliance states that an estimated two-thirds of school-based health centers have both a physical health provider and a mental health provider; as such this proximity can offer an opportunity for more expeditious care including screening and referrals for mental health concerns (Texas Care for Children, 2017). However, policy along with resources must follow in order to realize the benefits of the structure. Mental health professionals are commonly overtaxed with administrative duties and high student-to-counselor ratios that preclude them from being readily accessible to attend to students' mental health needs (Texas Care for Children, 2017). Of note, high schools sustaining a student to school counselor ratio of 250 students to 1 have demonstrated improved graduation and school attendance rates as well as reduced disciplinary events.

Importantly, most school-based health centers screen students for emotional concerns such as depression (76 %) and anxiety (71%) and an estimated 75% offer individual counseling for dating violence, substance use and suicide prevention (Texas Care for Children, 2017). School-based health centers can operate as catalysts and leaders in primary prevention endeavors to improve the health of school communities and engage students and staff in these efforts. Furthermore, school-based health centers have opportunities to participate in primary prevention pursuits that target the entire school thereby extending services beyond students to include adults in the community. An estimated 60% of school-based health centers identify that they serve populations other than the students in the school, nearly 84% serve students from other schools, about 66% serve family of student users, approximately 62% serve out-of-school youth, roughly 60% serve faculty/school personnel, and close to 36% serve other people in the community (School-Based Health Alliance, 2017).

Access to these services is specifically desirable in geographic areas and among populations that society disinvests in. For example, in Oregon 61% of school-based health centers are situated in primary care health professional shortage areas that are frequently rural and low-income. Of the 77 school-based health centers in Oregon, 19 serve chiefly students of color. Moreover, 52% of Oregon's school-based health centers clients are insured by Medicaid. Importantly they strive to practice integrating trauma-informed principles (Oregon School-Based Health Alliance, 2017). Interestingly, in Texas, State lawmakers displayed more attention to student mental health during the 2017 legislative session when they submitted a statute for the first time acknowledging the value of trauma-informed practice in schools in a multi-faceted student mental health bill (HB 3887). However, this bill was not successful in reaching a vote on the floor of the Texas House of Representatives (Texas Care for Children, 2017). Moreover, in Alameda County, California, school-based health centers are encompassing trauma-informed care to assist students to cope with the numerous stressors of community violence, family split-up, poverty and neglect, so students can flourish in school and life (School-Based Health Alliance, 2017). Some school-based health centers in East Oakland, California actually disseminate a school-wide screen to detect student's exposure to chronic stress. School-based health center staff establish initiatives to diminish the results of and foster resilience against trauma and toxic stress; some of these initiatives include trauma-focused support groups, healing circles, behavioral health consultations, and coordination of services (School-Based Health Alliance, 2017). Furthermore, several school-based health centers offer teacher workshops to support their understanding of how childhood adverse conditions frequently show up as learning problems in the schoolroom. Intentional steps have been implemented to expand these offerings with the California School-Based Health Alliance receiving a grant for $2 million from the San Francisco Foundation to team up with the Oakland Unified School District and Alameda County's Center for Healthy Schools and Communities to extend comparable advances to Oakland's entire production of school-based health centers (School-Based Health Alliance, 2017).

Importantly, students served in school-based health centers have exhibited improved educational and health outcomes, comprising higher grade point averages, decreased use of the emergency department, fewer hospital admissions, and reduced frequencies of drug and alcohol use. School-based health centers have also been associated with safe and supportive school climates as well as students having stronger bonds with their schools. These are favorable indicators, given that we have an estimated 2,000 school-based health centers operating nationwide (Health Resources and Services Administration, 2017). The National School-Based Health Care Census (2017) states that in their 2013–14 census of school-based health centers 2,315 supply services for students and communities in 49 of 50 states as well as the District of Columbia. There has been a 20% increase in the number of school-based health centers since the 2010–2011 Census, adding 385 new programs (School-Based Health Alliance, 2017). Most of these centers are located in traditional schools (66.6%) followed by community (10%), magnet (6.7%), vocation (6%), alternative (5%), charter (2.9%), and parochial/private (1.1%) (School-Based Health Alliance, 2017). Furthermore, an estimated 94% of school-based health centers are situated on school property, 3% are mobile health centers, 2.7 % are school-linked, and 0.2% are telehealth (School-Based Health Alliance, 2017).

In conclusion, this chapter highlights that trauma and its associated consequences are not waning and therefore it is an opportune time for health professionals to be aligned with more

11

COMMUNITY AND SOCIETAL TRAUMA-INFORMED INTERVENTIONS

Community and broader societal trauma-informed interventions are greatly influenced by micro-level processes including individual knowledge about ACEs as well as the values, culture, beliefs, laws and customs of those in power in the broader society. While exposure to trauma is pervasive in societies worldwide, traumatic experiences do not simply take place indiscriminately or in a vacuum; they are influenced by individual characteristics, family relationships, peer group relationships, community characteristics, and socio-political forces. Consequently, societal structure becomes embodied and as a result produces circumstances that often lead to trends in suffering which are greater among particular populations. Thus, this embodiment is a fluctuating macro-micro-macro process, and intrinsically an inevitable multilevel phenomenon.

Since people do not function in isolation of any of the ecological systems, macrosystem philosophies have significant effects on microsystem functioning. For instance, a philosophical system that regards families as private and difficulties within families, or with children, as personal responsibilities, is inclined to lack support services for families (Dowd, 2017). Dissimilarities, particularly economic ones, are considered as an outcome largely from personal choices. Conversely, a philosophical system of solidarity and mutual support is frequently revealed in institutional supports for families founded in the principle that affording supports for children and their families offers long-run advantages to the social good (Dowd, 2017). Thus, interventions that occur at the macrosystem level will engage with the cultural and subcultural foundations of thought and information on matters such as economic, political, educational, and legal domains. This is vital as the macrosystem indirectly conveys what form of social support is seen as appropriate through established social, economic, and political structures and processes having distinct effects on children and their families (Noffsinger, Pfefferbaum, Pfefferbaum, Sherrieb, & Norris, 2012). A system governed by a philosophy of private responsibility and non-intervention in families, alternatively, may offer negligible support and justify inequalities as privately produced instead of publicly structured (Dowd, 2017).

When developing interventions to address ACEs, using an ecological systems perspective along with a strengths-based underpinning (e.g., policies, practice approaches, and strategies that recognize and pull upon the strengths, possibilities, and resiliencies of youth, families, and communities) is paramount rather than the typical deficit and problem-focused approach, which underscores difficulties and pathology. Moreover, in addition to moving away from policy that focuses on individualizing problems and blaming, policy must aid the least privileged individuals in society. To more fully realize the effectiveness of a strengths-based approach, it needs to be supported by other policy initiatives that address structural difficulties that may contribute to the child's, family's, and community's circumstances.

As we strive to create a wholesome ecology that is well-functioning, our desire should be to see that people in the microsystem are systemically supported. This offers crucial structural and cultural support to the child, as well as to others who most immediately affect the person's well-being. Therefore, families and neighborhoods reciprocally reinforce positive development. This affords a safe and stimulating setting in which children can grow and be equipped to start school. But, when systems are in conflict, stress is created and it can become toxic and eventually situations can become traumatic; this can occur directly to the child or indirectly, through nonexistent support of their most vital interactions. As an illustration, if work and family exosystems of parents (e.g., work demands, ease of access to high quality child care, income support where needed) are in conflict, parents have challenges with affording time and quality nurturance provided to their children. Ultimately, this affects parental and family dynamics, and consequently impacts the child. Accordingly, the macrosystem of ideas and philosophies is significant as it relates to the operationalization of the entire ecosystem. In the end, a system of shared support and unity supports the idea that *all children are our children*, and looks after each young person in a child-centered, individually correct manner. Considering this, for example, a focus on a child that lacks attention to race and gender is a disservice as these factors generate structural and cultural difficulties especially in the US. Within our racialized society, for instance, the reality is that the social construction of race, and the beliefs and opportunities that come with it, are involved in every interaction in our society, affecting "life experiences, life opportunities, and social relationships" (Greer, 2017, p. 3). Moreover, differential supports for these children would mean the incorrect questions are being asked which is crucial since policy seeks to 'fix' what is considered a divergence from the norm versus exposing why structures, institutions, and policies continue to replicate inequality. As Dowd (2017) argues, the actual norms against which children of color have been assessed are white norms. This is illustrated in the fact that practically all child development theory and research has been either entirely or largely concentrated on white children. When interventions for ACEs are directed by policy for children it must use the voluminous data and substantial literature known about implicit bias, stereotypes, racism, and structural discrimination that challenge normative developmental possibilities; subsequently, the developmental model needs to be re-framed to take such factors into account (Dowd, 2017). Also, ACEs, other traumas, and our racialized society can be invisible to the eyes of health professionals who have not been exposed to them or those who have not been educated to perceive and effectively respond to them since the causes of an individual's or community's behaviors may be masked to the person who has good intentions of serving. To promote developmental equality or even developmental equity, interventions using models that are raced and gendered must be used to (a) recognize the structural and cultural barriers that are often encountered and (b) dismantle structures in the ecological systems that produce such disparate challenges, and employ systems that support children's rightful development.

Examples of interventions taking place at the exo-level and macro-level will be highlighted in this chapter such as (a) the larger community including state level initiatives, (b) the broader societal norms comprising coverage in the news media, (c) medical practice, (d) federal level initiatives encompassing the justice system, and (e) the need for interventions to ameliorate economic distress contributing to poverty and homelessness and the financial costs of ACEs.

Community

Community interventions that address ACEs and other exposures to trauma must be considerate of ecological context including community culture to effectively attend to the community's vulnerability and foster community healing by enhancing community assets. Attention to these areas is vital while community interventions focus on the individual as well as the entire community in order to develop resiliency. Importantly, one community intervention is not necessarily transferrable to every community context. This is evident because of the numerous and varied ecological features that must be taken into account. When communities have a broad assortment of resources and numerous opportunities for its members to affect community life, this is an idyllic setting for individuals to become resilient. Promoting the development of settings resembling this is or should be a categorical objective of community interventions to advance resilient functioning. As an illustration, exemplars of community interventions undertaken will be highlighted.

There are many states that have started to take intentional steps to intervene with ACEs. California recognizes that childhood trauma is having extensive effects on the state's education, public health, juvenile and criminal justice system, as well as youth's bodies, brains and future (Merck, 2018). To move efforts forward, the state developed the California Campaign to Combat Childhood Adversity in 2014. The three prevailing steps undertaken include (a) approval of a resolution to encourage evidence-based solutions to decrease childhood exposure to trauma along with financing preventive care and interventions (e.g. home visiting programs to promote health and well-being of families, instituting a 12-year age minimum for juvenile justice, and curbing removal of children from school) (b) development of an action plan and five major policy strategies to tackle childhood trauma in the California Legislature as well as (c) assembling a toolkit to aid other state advocates to replicate this initiative (Merck, 2018). The California Campaign to Combat Childhood Adversity similarly sought to assist other states formulate related advancements to tackle disparities and structural inequities in systems to preclude and respond to childhood adversity.

The toolkit offers language that can be used to scaffold discussion related to childhood adversity, identifiable goals and objectives, approaches to accomplish the objectives, and leading principles to enlighten the work. Material used in this toolkit was aligned with communication materials California Campaign to Combat Childhood Adversity applied when having conversations with policymakers and staffers during an earlier Policymaker Education Day. This material is also useful in preparing for preliminary and follow-up exchanges with elected representatives and their staffers (Merck, 2018).

Tonette Walker, the First Lady of Wisconsin, is a leader in the crusade to integrate trauma-informed policy across its state government to transform health care and communities. Her platform issue is supported through Fostering Futures, an organization that

TABLE 11.1 California Policy Strategies to Address Childhood Trauma (Merck, 2018)

Strategy	Description
Develop a trauma-informed workforce.	Promote inclusion of competency on trauma-informed approaches be included on professional licensure and certification standards. Encourage education on the undesirable effects of childhood adversity, along with how to foster protective factors and resilience.
Recruit and educate a diverse workforce.	Be intentional on constructing enticements to employ diverse services providers especially in communities that are exposed to childhood adversity more severely and deeply. Also, educate a diverse workforce on childhood adversity and trauma-informed methods.
Expand funding and access to deal with childhood adversity.	Increase subsidy and access to applicable and promising treatments and practices that focus on childhood adversity, particularly for communities that are exposed to high levels of childhood adversity.
Promote timely recognition of childhood adversity.	Push for early detection of childhood adversity along with effective and encouraging treatments and practices.
Raise public awareness and cultivate trauma-informed systems.	Champion for parents and caregivers as they strive to be productive and supportive adults for children. Support child and family serving systems and businesses to integrate trauma-informed methods into their policy and practice.

partners with the Wisconsin Department of Children and Families and several private associations to better identify, understand, and focus on the effects of trauma on the lives of children and families in Wisconsin (Bauerly, 2018; Luest, 2017). As a result of Walker's backing on this initiative, in 2014, Wisconsin became the first state in the United States to pass a joint resolution tackling early childhood adversity. In addition, this resolution called for state policy rulings to integrate ACEs science including theories of early childhood brain development and toxic stress, early adversity, and protective relationships. Moreover, the resolution indicated the preference of early intervention and financing of early childhood years as vital approaches to realize an enduring underpinning for a more thriving and justifiable state through investing in human capital (Bauerly, 2018). Although this resolution was set forth, it did not sanction new programs; it symbolized an essential legal tool for enhancing awareness about ACEs and delivered a focal agenda for state level decision-making (Bauerly, 2018). It was in 2016 that Governor Scott Walker charged state agencies in Wisconsin, specifically the Department of Veterans Affairs, the Department of Health Services Division of Public Health, the Wisconsin Economic Development Corporation, the Department of Health Services Children's Long-Term Supports, the Department of Corrections, the Department of Children and Families, and the Department of Workforce Development to take part in a learning collaborative headed by Fostering Futures to familiarize themselves with ACEs and to execute trauma-informed practices for their departmental personnel. Following the implementation of the learning collaborative, encouraging outcomes have been noted, for instance, the Economic Development Corporation observed a profound decrease in its voluntary attrition rate for its workers the first year these strategies were employed. Likewise, the Department of Justice has mobilized efforts with respect to improving community response to sexual attacks by employing a trauma-informed, person-centered approach. Similarly, the State Public Defender's Office not only integrated trauma-informed practices to help its staff along with its clients but also took part in research examining the influence of compassion fatigue (i.e., collective physical, emotional, and psychological outcomes developing from recurrent exposure to others' traumatic experiences) on its personnel and how to alleviate these effects. In the words of First Lady Walker, "The benefits of trauma informed-care reach far beyond the person affected, extending to the family, community, state, and even the nation" (Luest, 2017, ¶ 2). Walker's vision is that everyone regardless of positon (e.g., bus driver, to the lunch aide, to the school administrator, the governor, and even the president of the US) becomes trauma-informed and is aware of its meaning (Luest, 2017).

Change in mind

Collaboration across states and provinces has also been developed to address ACEs. For instance, Change in Mind, a project of the Alliance for Strong Families and Communities in alliance with the Robert Wood Johnson Foundation as well as the Palix Foundation's Alberta Family Wellness Initiative, display the powerful influence of the nonprofit sector to line up the science with the aim of inspiring systems to favorably affect outcomes across the life course. In North America both the US (10 members of the alliance) and Alberta, Canada (five non-governmental organizations of the alliance) took part in the initiative to instill, align, and accelerate recognized neuroscience breakthroughs regarding the effects of life-changing toxic stress into their community-based work (Jones & Olson, 2018). Using cutting-edge science to transform policies to address some of the most challenging social issues encountered by our communities is a major undertaking. Targeted attention was given to implanting research on brain science into organizational cultures, practices, and programs; leveraging scientific improvements in brain development to accelerate region and systems change; hastening systems change within a broader policy context; and adopting peer learning via a peer-based learning community model (Jones & Olson, 2018). Specific sites in the US leading in this initiative were diverse including (a) the Children's Home Society of Washington in Seattle, (b) East End House in Cambridge, Massachusetts, (c) Children and Families First in Wilmington, Delaware, (d) Wellspring Family Services in Seattle, (e) LaSalle School in Albany, New York, (f) the Children's Hospital of Wisconsin in Milwaukee, (g) The Family Partnership in Minneapolis, (h) KVC Health Systems in Olathe, Kansas, (i) the Family Service Association of San Antonio in San Antonio, and (j) the Martha O'Bryan Center in Nashville, Tennessee. In Canada, the particular sites involved comprised: (a) the Sheldon Kennedy Child Advocacy Centre in Calgary, (b) CASA Child, Adolescent, and Family Mental Health in Edmonton, (c) Big Brothers, Big Sisters of Calgary and Area in Calgary, (d) CUPS Health, Education, Housing in Calgary, and (e) the Boyle McCauley Health Centre in Edmonton (Jones & Olson, 2018). A developmental evaluation approach was a critical step in this initiative, using theories of change, and more is underway including monitoring, tracking, and mapping each site's development as well as identifying patterns of activity across organizational types and country contexts. This strategy differentiated Change in Mind from other ACEs and resilience programs (Jones & Olson, 2018).

Philadelphia ACE Task Force

Philadelphia, Pennsylvania, one of the poorest of the 10 most densely inhabited cities in the US, with the highest rate of deep poverty among large cities, has high levels of ACEs (37% of Philadelphians) according to results from an expanded ACEs assessment (Chilton, 2018). In essence, Philadelphia has become a trauma-organized city; that is, traumatic experiences have become normalized in the life of the community and have virtually been rendered invisible with its everyday occurrence. In 2015, the Philadelphia ACE Task Force joined alliance with a group of 14 communities from all over the nation via the Mobilizing Action for Resilient Communities (MARC) initiative. Organized by the Health Federation of Philadelphia and championed by the Robert Wood Johnson Foundation as well as the California Endowment, the MARC initiative has been essential in assisting the Philadelphia ACE Task Force to consider how the Philadelphia community can be a part of a developing national movement to foster a just, salubrious, and resilient world (Philadelphia ACE Project, 2019). Specifically, key priorities for the Philadelphia ACE Task Force include educating the community concerning ACEs, trauma, and resilience; understanding the useful interventions currently employed in Philadelphia to attend to childhood adversity and trauma; preparing the labor force with the knowledge and skills necessary to integrate trauma-informed practices into their work; and applying the Philadelphia Expanded ACE Data to enhance recognition of the effect of community-level adversities (Philadelphia ACE Project, 2019).

Other cross-sector collaboration has also prompted innovative community partnerships and trauma-informed interventions with programs of varied types. Examples include Healing Hurt People (a hospital-based program that assists young men injured in street violence and wards off revengeful violence), the Building Wealth and Health Network (infusing trauma-informed practices in the welfare system's education and training programs for caregivers of young children), and other youth programs offering protective along with growth-promoting relationships and safe spaces (Porch Light, The Village of Arts and Humanities, and Philly Young Playwrights) (Chilton, 2018).

Philadelphia is recognized as a national leader in trauma education holding numerous conferences to mobilize many organizations dedicated to healing children, families, and communities. However, regardless of how bold Philadelphia's programming is, the health and social service sectors have much work to do moving upstream to tackle the root sources of trauma—systemic neglect and ethnic, racial and gender discrimination (Chilton, 2018). To actually be effective, trauma-informed policymaking is requisite to enhance mobilization of trauma responsiveness. Meaningful action must occur at the city level and higher (Chilton, 2018).

Ultimately, the lasting effect of successful interventions depends on their being embedded in and known to more prevailing social settings and community contexts. Mindfulness to the prospects for safeguarding lasting effects and enduring transformations are essential characteristics of trauma-informed intervention design and management as well as developmental science with trauma-responsive interventions.

TABLE 11.2 Representative Agencies in Philadelphia That Have Moved from Knowledge to Action (Philadelphia CeaseFire, 2014; Trauma Informed Philanthropy, 2016)

Organization	Sector	Intervention
Children's Crisis Treatment Center	Behavioral health	Internal policy change from human resources to reimbursement policy along with engaging consumers and families in advisory and leadership capacities as well as committees; applied Sanctuary principles to services beyond residential behavioral health; strengths-based practices. Sanctuary certified.
Steven and Sandra Sheller 11th Street Family Health Services	Health care	Educated community advisory committee (CAC) members about brain architecture, the impact of stress, and ACEs. CAC then disseminated knowledge to neighborhood residents as ambassadors for the trauma-informed movement and as part of the Philadelphia ACE Task Force, and the local trauma-informed cross-sector network. Strong emphasis on community messaging and ACEs and trauma; Sanctuary certified.
Youth Sentencing and Reentry Project (YSRP)	Criminal Justice	YSRP partners with policy and advocacy organizations to drive broader systems change. Links with policy groups to advocate for legislative and regulatory action allowing the advocacy process to involve those with lived experience thus mitigating tokenizing and re-traumatizing YSRP's client-partners.
CeaseFire	Community violence intervention	Youth leadership and peer mediation program to interrupt gang violence in hot spots specifically in North Philadelphia; Cross sectional partners.

News media

The role of the media, specifically the news, plays an integral role as it relates to interventions for ACEs since traditional news outlets continue to be a main source of information for the preponderance of news consumers (Nixon, Somji, Mejia, Dorfman, & Quintero, 2015). News media can place ACEs on the public agenda, supporting local endeavors, enhancing consciousness and transmitting basic information (Han, 2017). The manner in which ACEs is talked about in the news affects the broader communities understanding and viewpoint both of the problem and of conceivable resolutions. If news reporting renders discussion on ACEs invisible or does not create links to the societal circumstances that promote childhood trauma, it minimizes the possibility for policymakers and the public to consider ACEs as urgent or acknowledge it as a problem that can be averted. It is important for the news media to relate the need for multilevel interventions to prevent and attend to ACEs and develop resilient communities which necessitate the involvement of many consisting of health care, criminal justice, education, and business (Nixon et al., 2015). Yet, the affiliations between these divisions and ACEs often lack prominence in the news, obfuscating reality that schools, industries and other participants have an essential role in stopping or addressing ACEs as well as their effects on individuals and communities. That said, the news media addressing ACEs could dissuade constructive engagement and bolster notions that ACEs is intractable if it conceals the interconnections amid ACEs and different divisions of our society. The broader social context in which ACEs take place, and the numerous individuals who are affected by them, can be described in narratives (e.g., abuse, neglect, violence) as well as in accounts in news arenas including business and education news, or in stories concerning any area that has a part in inhibiting or tackling ACEs.

In regards to schools, the news media can speak to the interconnections between ACEs and how it impacts a child's aptitude to learn, effecting scholastic accomplishments. Moreover, when children are exposed to ACEs, a rise in mental and behavioral health resources in schools will be needed to address increased disciplinary concerns, violent behavior including bullying, along with attendance issues. Furthermore, news media can disentangle the effects of retaliatory school discipline which exacerbate students' ACE exposure and instead promote restorative justice. Likewise, the news media can speak to the links between businesses and ACE-related effects impacting workers such as loss of productivity, increased health insurance and health care costs due to deteriorating health and mental health outcomes. What's more, media should highlight the benefits of intervening in these settings to promote both wellness and leadership development programs which can easily be integrated in the news. As well, developing emotional and social intelligence programs may well benefit all workers, particularly those who have been exposed to ACEs since these forms of intelligence interventions increase both emotional coping resources and social skills coping with adversity encountered in business environments.

Children are exposed to ACEs daily, and while exposure regarding ACEs is mounting, they are seldom mentioned in US news reporting (Han, 2017). They are generally remarked on in the context of incidents or initiatives endorsed by the health or social services areas, instead of, for instance, individually-focused accounts regarding particular situations of ACEs. This exemplifies a worthwhile opportunity for activists to discuss both prevention and intervention given that articles concerning programs or events to deal with ACEs are an inherent place to comment on how social and physical settings, consisting of governmental and organizational policies and practices can preclude or promote ACEs (Nixon et al., 2015). Moreover, when well-known and respected individuals have a platform and discuss ACEs, people give attention to what they have to say. For example, Oprah Winfrey recently learned about ACE science and she related "It blew my mind. It changed my life" (Caven, 2018, ¶ 3). She learned how organizations are employing a variety of ACE-informed approaches, such as trauma-informed care. Her insights in asking the following question is insightful, "You know some people talk about this cycle of poverty, the cycle of joblessness, homelessness, incarceration. Can those problems be solved without addressing trauma?" (Winfrey, 2018). Discussions with leading researchers such as Dr. Perry enable Oprah to now reflect on *what happened to people who harm others*. It is real that trauma leads to trauma in our families, communities, as well as in the world. While many devastating events are occurring in our world especially as relates to guns, placing resources toward gun control as well as mental health is needed; however, Oprah also asserts that we must explore the *hole in the soul* and provide services to people in need (Noonan, 2018).

According to Noonan (2018), communications director for the Institute for Attachment and Child Development, some coverage of ACEs in the news media including Oprah's interview has illustrated that:

- Not all clinicians really understand ACEs the way they think they do; however key leaders in ACE efforts such as Dr. Bruce Perry, Daniel Siegel, Dr. Sandy Bloom, and Bessel van der Kolk get it. Their work has been integral to constructing treatment models.

- ACEs affect the brain in a critical way, especially when exposure strikes during critical early stages of life. There is a realization that it is not simply a stage that individuals 'get over' or 'outgrow' as per the belief of many individuals. More accurately, ACE exposure necessitates early and effective professional intervention.

- Because ACEs during the critical early developmental years hinders development, the Diagnostic and Statistical Manual of Mental Disorders, 5th Edition should use the term developmental trauma rather than reactive attachment disorder. Given that individuals who have experienced ACEs often become cognitively trapped in those early years, using terminology that resonates more accurately can help clinicians begin to identify and support the person's healing process through effective treatment.

- ACEs are a major issue for our culture as childhood trauma does not solely affect children; these children are haunted throughout adulthood and subsequently. These children enter schools and often prisons and experience mental and behavioral health issues. Left unchecked and having access to guns brings about significant devastation. It's time to wake up!

- Philanthropic organizations who strive to aid those whom are on the margins of society often are mistaken by focusing on limited areas. While those who are fraught with many needs require education, healthy living, housing, and adequate employment, we must also assist them with what Oprah calls *the hole in their soul*. That is, healing work on their trauma must occur in order for these individuals to lead healthier lives. Similarly, placing those affected by ACEs in residential treatment centers and working solely on behavior modification approaches will not necessarily work on their trauma exposure. These individuals must have a relationship-focused milieu along with attachment experts to help creäte positive change.

- Parents and care takers of children with developmental trauma need help to effectively care for their children however, they tend to get criticized and shamed when they seek help. They live through these challenges every day yet family, friends, other professionals (e.g., clinicians, educators, and case managers), and policy makers discount their experiences. Shockingly, sometimes they are even blamed for their children's difficulties.

- We are lacking health professionals competent in dealing with children who are exposed to childhood trauma and what to do about it. As well, there is a dearth of resources allocated to address the issue worldwide. While individuals have long been informed about the implications of childhood trauma steps are needed to appropriately educate clinicians to effectively diagnose and treat it.

- Co-morbid mental illnesses are common among children who have experienced developmental trauma. Those who inflict childhood trauma tend to also have a history of trauma combined with mental illness which heightens risk for transgenerational childhood trauma and genetic mental health concerns. However, most clinicians have a challenging time untangling, and consequently diagnosing and treating, these various issues.
- Attachment is difficult for children with developmental trauma since they often get stuck in 'survival mode,' thus doing everything they can against forming attachment while that is precisely what is needed to support them on their journey to healing. Lacking appropriate intervention, these children with developmental trauma employ manipulation and alarming behaviors to alienate those who attempt to form any type of close connection. Simply having caring and loving adults, be they family-related, foster, or adoptive adults, in their lives is insufficient; this does not effectively address childhood trauma. However, this environmental climate is important as well as appropriately trained professionals in addition to resources needed to prevent propagating the effects of trauma.

Han (2017) also addresses the need for broader sectors of the community beyond health care to speak up and speak out about ACEs. All segments need to attend to the link between health equity and the discussion of ACEs. Relevant interventions that the news can implement to support proactive measures regarding ACEs include:

(a) Adopting prevention as a normative part of the conversation with the public, helping them to think about the various approaches communities can preclude childhood trauma by offering explicit detailed examples which helps to defy the conception that childhood trauma is too overwhelming and intractable to address and it also affords blueprints for other people to carry out prevention work in their own communities;

(b) Developing capacity among leaders from an array of areas to converse effectively about ACEs from their perspectives and foster coalitions of leaders to co-create a shared vision for advocacy. Creating media advocacy training is also key so news personnel can express knowledge about childhood trauma effectively. As an illustration, having greater numbers of teachers, academic administrators, corporate owners and community members who are cognizant of and interested in ACEs and can speak about solutions, allows for more people to enhance the profile of ACEs as a serious and preventable matter for the entire community; and

(c) Pointing out race and equity concerns and the community context of childhood trauma given that racism, poverty, community violence as well as other structural inequities are indistinguishably related to childhood trauma. Prevention and successful interventions can only occur when communities make trauma visible and while the news seldom composes links between childhood trauma and structural inequities, news reporters can make this evident in their storytelling. In addition to unapologetically talking about race and structural inequity, we must too have discourse concerning hope to help move attention to the broader social change required to produce and uphold trauma-informed and trauma-free communities (Han, 2017).

As noted by Nixon, Rodriguez, Han, Mejia, and Dorfman (2017), pertinent lines of query that can advance meaningful interventions regarding childhood trauma include: (a) Do all children obtain similar chances for attaining optimal health? If not, why? (b) Which children in the community are at greater risk of exposure to childhood trauma and why? (c) Make visible environmental, structural and community-level circumstances that are inflicting trauma on children? And what needs to be done to ease these circumstances? (d) Ascertain where other communities have been victorious in addressing comparable problems and determine how communities impacted by trauma can leverage resources and skills to conquer the problem. As a final point, who can and should be considered responsible and accountable to make certain that childhood trauma is addressed in an effective manner? Reporters who take their ethical sense of duty seriously to function as advocates on behalf of the public are positioned well to champion for change. This aforementioned line of query can have significant implications for childhood trauma-related issues.

Medical practice

Medical practices encounter individuals of all ages and even though there is a high prevalence of ACE-related traumatic events impacting people with undesirable health and health system costs, clients and clinicians do not commonly speak about these issues during medical encounters (e.g., primary care). Abaek, Kinn, and Milde (2017) report that many health professionals believe they are unequipped and lack resources (organizational culture and/or system attributes) required to effectively attend to the needs of individuals exposed to high levels of ACE-related traumatic events. This is comparable to moving through a minefield devoid of clear plans for safe passages or tools to neutralize mines. Furthermore, clinicians fear that their efforts to support could further injure the patient they are working with; this is analogous to walking a person into an unidentified minefield and risk activating unseen mines (i.e., fear of exacerbating the situation). When individuals confront ACE-related traumatic events, they tend to experience emotional distress that brings forth avoidance patterns, similar to how getting into a minefield with a threat to harm producing fear and avoidance (Abaek et al., 2017).

Medical professionals such as primary care providers (e.g., adult or family nurse practitioners, physician assistants, pediatricians, family practice physicians) are well-positioned to change the way the general public responds to individuals exposed to significant ACEs. There is increased knowledge in understanding the importance of early life experiences for individual's health throughout the life course, specifically people who experience ACEs during childhood or adolescence who typically have greater physical and behavioral health issues as adults compared to those who are not exposed to ACEs and ultimately elevated levels of early death, therefore health care providers must act. This is a necessity since 20%–50% of adult individuals report sexual or physical abuse and 44% report childhood physical, sexual, or emotional abuse (Weinreb et al., 2010). Interestingly, in spite of this developing concern, primary care providers seldom screen clients for ACEs, or assess the effect of childhood experiences on their well-being. This was illustrated in research conducted by Weinreb et al. (2010) with physicians and Kalmakis, Chandler, Roberts, and Leung (2016) with nurse practitioners in primary care medical settings. Weinreb learned that less than one-third of primary care physicians screened for childhood trauma or abuse (Weinreb et al., 2010) and

Kalmakis et al. (2016) revealed comparable outcomes with 33% of the nurse practitioners screening for adverse events. To better understand these challenges, this section examines provider background and vicarious trauma, especially implications when a provider practices in a trauma-informed manner, interprofessional collaboration, and trauma-informed supervision/coaching.

Provider background and vicarious trauma

Similar to other adults, health care providers are exposed to substantial levels of childhood and adult trauma. Thus, a personal history of abuse could affect not only health care providers' own health status, it may well affect how they screen, react and care for clients with childhood or adult trauma. While medical settings seldom encourage health care providers to examine and understand their own trauma histories, it is critical to effectively provide trauma-informed care and promote awareness to initiate appropriate interventions with their clients (Raja, Hasnain, Hoersch, Gove-Yin, & Rajagopalan, 2015). Moreover, when healthcare providers are survivors of traumatic events, they may be apprehensive about talking about these issues not wanting to retrigger their own feelings (Raja et al., 2015). Candib, Savageau, Weinreb, & Reed (2012) report that health care providers have comparable exposure to trauma to the general population. For example, their rate of witnessing violence between parents is 11.6% compared to 13% in a national survey. Similarly, their rate of childhood sexual abuse is 21.9% for females and 11.1% for male health care providers compared with those in the original ACE study and a national metanalysis—25% of women and 16% of men (ACE) and of 30%– 40% for females and 13% for males (national metanalysis) respectively (Candib et al., 2012). Intimate partner violence was the only area of trauma that demonstrated no correlation between healthcare providers and the general population with 9.3% for women and 4.9% for men compared with 25% women, 11% men in the general population (Candib et al., 2012).

Interestingly, even among health care providers with exposure to trauma, gender has been shown to be an independent predictor of screening. Specifically, female physicians are frequently more prone to screen for childhood abuse histories than their male counterparts. This may sensitize female physicians to the effects of traumas and lead them to be more confident with regularity of screening for trauma. Having been predisposed to trauma, healthcare providers themselves could limit examination of or diminish the significance of such events or, instead, be provoked and persuaded to screen more than they otherwise would (Weinreb, et al., 2010). Educating health care providers to recognize the implications of their own personal histories is important since these experiences can impact their practice.

Additionally, a healthcare provider's chronic exposure to clients suffering can contribute to vicarious trauma resulting in maladaptive responses including compassion fatigue and professional burnout. Healthcare providers must consider their risk for vicarious trauma which relates to deleterious changes that can come about for a health care provider that specifically changes their viewpoints about themselves and others, as well as their worldview (see Figure 11.1).

Vicarious trauma surfaces when a health care provider has contact with individuals who have experienced traumatic events which cause powerful emotional reactions that may arise when healthcare providers listen to descriptions of traumatic events (Raja et al., 2015). Given the ubiquity of trauma, it is increasingly understood that health care providers' stress,

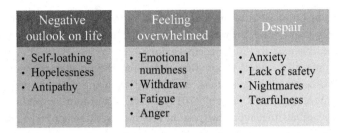

FIGURE 11.1 Signs and Symptoms of Vicarious Trauma

frequently labeled as vicarious, is actually associated with providers' own trauma exposures and the degree to which individuals' experiences allow these exposures to surface to the forefront of the provider's mind. Unearthing ways to recognize these dynamics, and to create a work atmosphere that is a healing place for health care providers and clients, is important. This is an essential aspect of organizational climate in trauma-informed care. Self-awareness and self-care among healthcare providers is also critical in order to alleviate the effects of vicarious trauma they experience. Empathy is grounded in self-awareness and empathic communication becomes almost impractical when a health care provider becomes devastated by the emotional facets of day-to-day practice. Strategies that can be implemented to mitigate vicarious trauma and create positive energy can be viewed in Figure 11.2.

It is important for these providers to pay special attention to the indications of compassion fatigue and professional burnout. Compassion fatigue reduces a provider's ability or desire to be empathic and bear their clients' pain. Thus, compassion fatigue contrasts vicarious traumatization because it is a more universal expression largely depicting a professional's experience of emotional and physical exhaustion because of the protracted use of empathy. It does not require direct relations with traumatized individuals (Sansbury, Graves, & Scott, 2015) and tends to be located in combination with other bureaucratic obstacles that cause work-related stressors. Importantly, compassion fatigue is not restricted to professionals who perform trauma work and considers other factors implicated in an enduring demand for being empathetic. Healthcare providers who suffer from compassion fatigue experience isolation, vulnerability, helplessness and confusion. Compassion fatigue can be minimized for health care providers if they do not (a) disregard their own self-care, (b) evade working on their own trauma, and (c) have high work stressors. Once identified and effective interventions

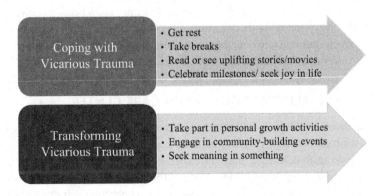

FIGURE 11.2 Coping and Transforming Vicarious Trauma (Jacksonville University, 2018)

implemented, compassion fatigue can dissolve with treatment. The very empathy that frequently motivates health care providers to enter the healing profession can also, if not acknowledged and planned for, make them victims.

Professional burnout, a gradual progression of feeling disconnected from meaningful relationships in response to prolonged stress, is depicted by being drained, unproductive, and having nothing more to give (Raja et al., 2015). In effect, burnout contributes to the extinguishment of the embers that represent passion for the healthcare providers work, to levels not explicable by duration of time worked. There are elevated levels of burn out among professionals world-wide; however, in the US, physicians appear to have the most elevated levels of all the professions, with nurses trailing close behind (Moffic, 2016). Medical students and residents appear to have escalating levels of burnout as their professional training advances (Moffic, 2016). Importantly, psychological, emotional, and/or physical exhaustion are commonplace manifestations of burnout. Also, four stages of burnout typically seen include: (a) physical and emotional exhaustion; (b) shame and doubt; (c) cynicism and callousness; and (d) failure, helplessness, and collapse (Avillion & Hamilton, 2018).

To mitigate undesirable manifestations of burnout, vicarious trauma, compassion fatigue and symptoms of traumatic stress, health care providers would benefit from individual protective factors (e.g., resolution of personal issues, on-going training, supervision, favorable physical, social, emotional and spiritual self-care, and robust moral principles of practice) and organizational protective factors (viewing the dilemma as group-wide versus individual focused; fostering open communication; solution-oriented rather than victim blaming; acceptance of stressors as genuine concerns; providers being backed using clear, direct, communication in a way that is complimentary and displays both commitment and affection) against these issues, including trauma-informed practices. Both of these factors can serve to be invaluable and promote improved organizational functioning and more effective practice with clients. Trauma-informed care underscores safety in discussing trauma for both providers and clients. With trauma-informed care, education occurs by recognizing the prevalence of violence that arises across the life course, including in the professional domain, and emphasizes the importance of using employee assistance programs and other resources. Discourse related to trauma and violence also makes more obvious often implicit concerns regarding compassion fatigue and vicarious trauma. Consequently, this allows dialogue about the provider's emotional well-being. Raja et al. (2015) state that providers should practice trauma-stewardship, part of trauma-informed care, which encompasses caring for the patient devoid of the provider assuming the patient's struggles. For health care providers this entails being mindful of reactions to challenging clients; appreciating that clients can become distressed or re-traumatized because of healthcare experiences and provider behaviors; and intentionally arranging for appropriate self-care by providers to afford optimal care to all clients (Raja et al., 2015).

BOX 11.1 CASE ILLUSTRATION: HEALTHCARE CENTER

In a large midwest city there is a health care center in a community that is very diverse, racially and ethnically. A large percentage of the population struggles to make ends meet financially. A white middle-aged male has directed the center for a decade, and the management staff is also primarily white. None of the management group lives within the community served. There are policies and procedures within the center that clients have difficulty complying with. One example is that there are requirements that all appointments be scheduled several days in advance; another is that the center closes each day at 4:30pm. The director, based on his experiences in a former position, largely set the policies and they have not undergone revision in years. The staff of the center is under time pressure and is rarely able to take time for lunch or breaks. The staff's meeting agendas are set by the director and are largely poorly attended. The staff complains that issues they have brought up such as the policies around appointment scheduling and the center hours have been ignored. Discontent is brewing and staff are beginning to form groups that are delineated around racial differences. There have been more absences of staff and patient care errors have increased.

Two staff members recently attended a conference on trauma-informed principles as they apply to the whole organization. The conference included issues of power, control and the unhealthy parallels that can develop in stressed organizations among leadership, staff and the community members served. The information resonated with the health center staff that attended and they have suggested that the director consider bringing the conference speaker to the center for a consultation. The director surprisingly agrees. In preparation for the consultation consider the following:

Discussion questions:

- Who would you suggest the consultant meet with in order to understand the issues in the organization?
- What are the norms reflected in the organization and who set them?
- Does it seem that community members have had a voice in determining the health center's policies?
- What would you suggest as a process to assist the staff to understand the culture and needs of the community served?
- What are some obstacles to building a trauma-informed organization do you identify?

  - At the level of client care?
  - At the level of staff care?
  - At the level of leadership?

- Can you identify signs of professional burnout in the staff?
- What are the essential issues around power and control that need to be addressed for this organization to implement trauma-informed practices?
- What seeds of opportunity for change can you identify at the center?

Interprofessional collaboration

Interprofessional collaboration, when diverse professional groups function together to positively influence health care among health care providers, is crucial when engaging clients exposed to trauma, which has adverse implications for cognitive, physical, and social development (Essen, Freshwater, & Cahill, 2015). Raja et al. (2015) further denote that interprofessionality moves beyond the bringing together of multiple professions delivering individual care to comprise cohesive, mutually dependent/supporting, and complementary working, while collaboration manifests as an interpersonal process where structuring of collective action occurs. Interprofessional collaboration permits clients to take advantage of being able to see various providers in a single appointment. It also allows health care professionals to gain an appreciation and understanding of professional roles and responsibilities of their fellow colleagues which supports effective management of clients who do disclose a trauma history (Raja et al., 2015). While interprofessional collaborative practice is the desired model when caring for persons impacted by trauma especially with its key elements of accessibility, collaborative structures and patient-centeredness we must also acknowledge the challenges of the model to support its success. Specifically, McWhinnie (2017) classified six obstacles to interprofessional collaboration which consist of "culture, self-identity, role clarification, decision-making, communication, and power dynamics" (p. 25). When bringing together professionals of different disciplines, power dynamics can play a huge role, particularly when historical power roles are inclined towards partiality with decision-making. Furthermore, decision-making itself can be problematic when professionals lack understanding or respect for roles held by their colleagues (McWhinnie, 2017).

Depending on the professional background and competence of the interprofessional health care members, external resources may be needed if the traumatized patient spontaneously discloses. If clients do extemporaneously reveal a trauma history, providers should be careful about probing deeply into the psychological background of clients, if they lack trauma training. Rather, these health care providers should be respectful and address the primary complaint for the current visit. For instance, if a woman conveys that she has been sexually abused in the past, which is producing anxiety at her visit, the healthcare provider can thank her for disclosing the information, inquire how they can make her more relaxed at the office visit, and extend her appropriate resources and referrals, if necessary (Raja et al., 2015).

This practice allows the healthcare provider an opportunity to recognize the patient's history while not traversing the limits of their professional competence. Healthcare providers must also regard the desires of those afflicted by trauma specifically with regard to reporting abuse when reporting is not legally required (Raja et al., 2015). Interprofessional collaboration can provide timely intervention and ensure continuity of care (Raja et al., 2015). Consideration of cultural diversity must also be taken into account when trauma-related interventions and access to appropriate referral services across systems is a goal. Experiences of trauma shape a patient's thoughts, feelings, beliefs, and worldview, as well as their cultural responses to services and treatment (Clervil & DeCandia, 2013). Similarly, it is just as significant to acknowledge that the cultural values of health care providers and medical systems have an influence on how services are delivered and accessed. Given that trauma has distinctive meanings across cultures and healing from trauma occurs within one's own cultural beliefs, health care providers and medical systems must have the capacity to operate effectively within the context of the cultural beliefs, behaviors, and needs indicated by survivors of trauma and their communities (Clervil & DeCandia, 2013). Ultimately, a trauma-informed approach to care is ideally culturally sensitive, allowing trauma survivors to reestablish both a sense of self as well as connection to their communities; presents an environment of mutual learning and assistance, respectful interactions, authentic partnerships in care provided; and allows providers to understand the role of cultural and linguistic differences related to their effect on service provision (Clervil & DeCandia, 2013). To that end, interprofessional collaboration has the potential to strengthen largescale endeavors to foster emotional support and meaningful relationships that is fundamental to healing of trauma survivors.

Trauma-informed supervision

Supervision is frequently the prime conduit for (a) educating and training staff, (b) supporting and integrating concepts into day-to-day practice, (c) ongoing assessment of workload needs, (d) providing space where staff can discuss work successes and challenges, as well as (e) reflecting on skills needed to improve their work (Guarino, Clervil, & Beach, 2014). However, "trauma-informed supervision is a lens through which the supervisor works and involves engaging the 'principles that guide trauma-informed practice, safety, trustworthiness, choice, collaboration, and empowerment'" (Varghese, Quiros, & Berger, 2018, p.1). Trauma-informed supervision brings together knowledge regarding trauma and supervision, and places emphasis on unique features of the interrelationship that exists related to the trauma, the clinician, as well as the setting in which the work is presented (Berger & Quiros 2014). Importantly, trauma-informed supervision has been identified as a key protective factor since it can operate as a safeguard against vicarious trauma; thus, trauma responses activated in clinicians due to working with traumatized clients implies that in trauma practice, it would be beneficial to engage in consistent forms of supervision (Berger & Quiros, 2014). This is critical because among helping professionals many may be unconscious and uninformed concerning the effect of trauma work, with regard to how it produces gradual changes in a person's assessment of the world and others (Wilson, 2016). Without trauma-informed supervision, helping professionals who have extensive and sustained exposure to trauma through their clients can acquire maladaptive coping processes, for example hypervigilance or isolation, which establishes an emotional barrier (Hunt, 2018).

Paralleling values of trauma-informed direct practice, fundamental to trauma-informed supervision is establishing a supervisory milieu that encourages emotional and physical safety, trustworthiness, preference, collaboration, and empowerment (Varghese et al., 2018). Encouraging the formation of such a milieu are individual characteristics of the supervisee as well as the supervisor, the quality of the supervisory relations, and organizational features. Preferably, a trauma-informed supervisor elicits a supervisee's experience and offers guidance. An integral component of trauma-informed supervision is acknowledgement of sociocultural aspects of supervision as it relates to race, ethnicity, and culture given that these aspects affect and shape the supervisory relationship (Hall & Spencer, 2017; Varghese et al., 2018). For example, if a supervisor lacks skill to engage their supervisee and inquire about their identities or experiences with race, ethnicity or culture, they can be in jeopardy of having a superficial relationship, leading the supervisee to withdraw or limit engagement in sharing. Therefore, a level of cultural proficiency is required; for instance, simply presuming that a dark-toned supervisee identifies as African American instead of, let's say, Dominican inhibits the supervisor from considering the lens by which the supervisee sees the world, which can influence how the supervisee practices. Disregarding the intricacy of the supervisee's distinctive experiences of race and ethnicity in the US context, including how individuals see themselves and are perceived by others, is essential to having an effective trauma-informed supervisory relationship (Watkins, 2014). Phillips, Parent, Dozier, and Jackson (2016) argue that the intensity of discussions about race, ethnicity, and culture along with other social identities leads to reduced levels of (a) role conflict, (b) role ambiguity, but (c) fervent supervisory working relationships connected to rapport and effectiveness of centering on clients. Nevertheless, research has demonstrated that supervisors typically disregard or evade conversations about race, ethnicity and culture due to the supervisor's personal discomfort or limited proficiency with these issues (Varghese et al., 2018). That said, not taking this information into consideration is not a benign practice; distinct ethnic groups should not be combined to establish a monolithic account of Blackness (Varghese et al., 2018).

Likewise, supervisors should also intentionally engage in conversations pertaining to power and privilege, aid with the supervisee's development of multicultural knowledge and competence, practice culturally-sensitive interventions during supervision, and undertake self-assessment of their own identity (Varghese et al., 2018). If these multifaceted elements of identity are overlooked, there will likely be impending detrimental effects for the supervisory relationship that impacts processes and outcomes. Tackling issues of power is key in the supervisory experience, considering evidence of racial and cultural connections influencing all aspects of trauma exposure; additionally, positions of power across gender, race, class, or ethnoreligious identity influence discourse (Quiros & Berger, 2015). This is markedly germane to the situation of trauma-informed supervision, since it is rooted within a structural hierarchy of power and matters of diversity and social justice are pertinent within this exchange.

This section has highlighted the relevance of trauma-informed supervision for supervisees, to limit the chances of becoming overinvolved and to support healthy relationship development to preclude excessive preoccupation with patient issues due to trauma exposure. Implementation of effective self-care is critical for both the supervisee and supervisor. Dialogue about trauma-informed supervision must also take on a sociopolitical lens to acknowledge supervisor's and supervisee's exposure to traumatic situations because of their social connections and social identities they are linked with. As well, assessing how these are enacted in their supervisory interaction is key. Along with the general concepts highlighted above regarding trauma-informed supervision, structural features (e.g., race, gender, power mechanisms) must be transparent and integrated into this relationship in meaningful ways.

Federal initiatives—the justice system

Trauma-informed practice originally acquired footing in human and mental health service areas but has lately been included by a wide array of sectors at multiple levels of government (Becker-Blease, 2017). For instance, federal initiatives including the White House's My Brother's Keeper and the Department of Justice's Defending Childhood Taskforce provide foundational efforts where the federal government could be the vanguard for development of standards of care for detection, assessment, interventions, safeguarding, and other vital services for children exposed to trauma, in addition to the development of protocols for examining the quality in these areas (Listenbee et al., 2012).

My Brother's Keeper is a federal initiative sponsored by President Obama in 2014 which provides the nation with an action-oriented program to advance outcomes for boys and men of color (Purtle & Lewis, 2017). Bold recommendations are to (a) tackle the systemic barriers confronting one of the nation's most vulnerable populations with trauma exposure with an extraordinary opportunity for the government to establish the framework and pace of change and (b) challenge the private sector, philanthropy, and community leaders to unite to realize collective impact. Significantly, trauma-informed social, emotional, physical and mental health supports are endorsed including in juvenile justice (Philadelphia Higher Education Network for Neighborhood Development, 2014). For instance, there is at least one My Brother's Keeper Community in each of the 50 states, as well as Puerto Rico and the District of Columbia. Furthermore, My Brother's Keeper Communities are located in 19 Tribal Nations. Considering communities that have made steep commitments, in April 2016 New York was the earliest among the states to subsidize a statewide venture in the My Brother's Keeper initiative by means of $20 million in funds. What's more over 140 Local Action Summits have occurred and greater than100 local action plans have either been publicized or are underway with community, charitable and commercial partners, faith leaders, and youth (My Brother's Keeper, 2016).

Also, the Department of Justice's Defending Childhood Taskforce introduced by Attorney General Eric Holder took effect in September 2010, with the purpose of collective investment nationally to protect children from exposure to trauma, in healing families and communities, and in allowing all children to envision and assert a secure, creative, and productive future (Listenbee et al., 2012; Purtle & Lewis, 2017). Fifty-six recommendations were derived from the Taskforce's work and listed within categories in these six chapters:

- *Chapter 1—Ending the Epidemic of Children Exposed to Violence*

  o Introductory recommendations are given and a summary of the problem is highlighted,

- *Chapter 2—Identifying Children Exposed to Violence and Chapter 3—Treatment and Healing of Exposure to Violence*

  o Presents recommendations that help to confirm reliable recognition, screening, and assessment of children subjected to trauma and the support, treatment, and services required to attend to their needs,

- *Chapter 4—Creating Safe and Nurturing Homes and Chapter 5—Communities Rising Up Out of Violence*

  o Concentrates on prevention and the need for effective incorporation of prevention, intervention, and resilience throughout systems,

- *Chapter 6—Rethinking Our Juvenile Justice System*

  o Appeals to the need for novel approaches to juvenile justice which recognizes that the great majority of youth in the system have been subjected to trauma and calls for the prioritization of services which can encourage their healing (Defending Childhood Initiative, 2013; Listenbee et al., 2012).

These recommendations endorse that change is capable of occurring and taking place with intentionality, in a timely manner, affecting governmental and community platforms at every level. Families should also be encouraged to unite in broader community efforts to join in with safeguarding and healing children who are endangered by trauma. While this should be a collective effort, this has not been realized as a nation. Not only are children harmed; lack of effective interventions often lead them to come in contact with the justice system (Listenbee et al., 2012).

There is growing awareness that both male and female justice involved youth are affected by trauma. Branson, Baetz, Horwitz, and Hoagwood (2017) state that approximately 70–90% of youth offenders have been subjected to one or more types of trauma (e.g., elevated rates of abuse, exposure to school or community violence, and witnessing household). Youth in the justice system with earlier trauma exposure and/or symptoms of post-traumatic stress disorder are a markedly susceptible population to have greater rates of recidivism, co-occurring disorders, drop-out, and suicide attempts compared to those in the general population (Branson et al., 2017; Steinberg & Lassiter, 2018). Moreover, rates rise as participation in the system escalates (Steinberg & Lassiter, 2018). Substance Abuse and Mental Health Services Administration's National Center for Trauma-Informed Care offers education, consultation, outreach, technical assistance, and resources to adopt a change to trauma-informed care with justice systems. For example, they made recommendations for modifications in education practices, furniture, and programming with their day-to-day operations. These modifications were intended to foster safety and a culture to support healing while evading avoidable power struggles. Some clear illustrations include approaching all youth from a perspective of universal trauma precautions. Also, undertaking a stance that all youth encountered in the justice system has a past trauma history; likewise, considering youth's emotional responses and behavior through a trauma lens (Steinberg & Lassiter, 2018).

Lastly, Garbarino (2017) argues that policy and practice recommendations are warranted in the justice system due to high levels of ACEs. These recommendations are warranted for several reasons. Specifically, it allows discussions to be grounded in justice versus the notion of choice. Having a belief that a killer has rendered bad choices, the underpinning for the criminal justice system, is one thing; however, do the 10 ACE items actually exemplify bad choices from a child? Do these children truly elect to amass the risk factors, trauma, and toxic stress appraised by the 10 ACE questions? Similarly, determining a developmental context before any assessment of personal liability ought to be a requirement at each location in a person's path through the criminal justice system. Secondly, employing ACE scores for youth provides a base for the entire courtroom dialogue in social reality. It also dismisses unwarranted judgments or false understandings of what is essential in sentencing. This is because, too often, a prosecutor will try to reject the significance of an offender's history of toxic stress and trauma with statements like, *many youths have horrific childhoods, what's the problem with this child?* Nevertheless, if a child has an elevated ACE score (of 8, 9, or 10), more than a generic childhood was experienced. That is, this youth had a childhood worse than 999 of 1000 youth in the US and this represents a powerful mitigating element when considering a penalty. Florida has taken intentional steps with judicial training, now making this prominent with understanding the effects of emerging ACEs research. Lastly, placing emphasis on cumulative childhood adversity and trauma grounds the justice system in developmental psychology and public health (Garbarino, 2017). Recognizing that ACE scores explain 65% of the difference in suicide attempts, 55% of the difference in substance abuse, 30% of the deviation in violent behavior, and 45% of the disparity in depression makes apparent the developmental importance of adversity, toxic stress, and trauma (Garbarino, 2017). More significantly, it speaks to the need for the justice system to take on a trauma-informed lens in sentencing judgments.

In conclusion, when reflecting on federal-related interventions, especially regarding the justice system, it is essential that an entree to trauma-informed therapeutic interventions is provided prior to any enduring judgments regarding their destiny. Implementation of developmental science is requisite. Supporting the rehabilitation and transformation of youth across the lifespan is important considering the immaturity of their brain and the plasticity of adult brains (Garbarino, 2017). Therapeutic interventions that aid with establishing a safe environment and avoid added traumatic factors is important to empower youth to recover from emotional and behavioral difficulties caused by trauma; this approach is key for youth, their families and communities, as well as personnel in the justice system who work with them. Meaningful interventions that address these issues within communities support development of a safer and healthier society.

Economic system

Economic systems are implicated when people do not have enough money; business and economic professionals have discovered that child development has a profound impact on the economic health of a community. Specifically, ACEs are often associated with different levels of economic resources. Within the US, one of the top most common ACEs is economic hardship. An estimated one-third of children in West Virginia have faced economic hardship, compared to one-fifth of children in Minnesota, New Hampshire, and North Dakota (Sacks & Murphey, 2018). As a macro-level force, the economic system influences the nature and frequency of trauma exposure and shapes the context in which individuals experience and react to them. This section will examine the relevance of providing interventions associated with ACEs and poverty, homelessness, as well as the financial costs of ACEs.

Poverty

Child poverty is the most pressing public health issue facing our world including the US and the United Kingdom (Hughes & Tucker, 2018; Mansour & Curran, 2016). Halfon (2016) states that poverty is formed in the very structure of our present economic reality; it adversely affects nearly every marker of child well-being and touches more than 1 in 5 children. Poverty is also a potent reinforcing factor in cumulative ACEs and consequent toxic stress associated with harmful health outcomes in adulthood (Hughes & Tucker, 2018). Child poverty is more than insufficiencies in income, resources, or services; this perspective is lacking since it does not acknowledge the complex nascent nature of poverty along with deep drivers that bring about ostensibly robust forces of deprivation and marginalization (Hughes & Tucker, 2018). Social ecology inherently causes poverty as a form of complex adaptive system; this lens also recognizes the numerous networks of social, economic, and cultural mechanisms that are independently and collectively changing, self-organizing and revealing nascent properties. Being poverty-stricken is linked with so many childhood adversities that it should be deemed an ACE in itself, more prevalent and persistent than all other ACEs.

Child poverty is often higher in single-parent families, and the single parent experiences a hardship in striving to accomplish roles of two parents. The poverty encountered by these children and families lacks uniformity; select populations encounter challenging times for short periods (situational poverty) while others suffer chronic poverty (generational poverty). Moreover, there may be those whose greatest hardship is scarce financial resources, whether limited income to address day-to-day expenditures or the essential resources (investments, a home) to move forward. Some individuals economic difficulties are compounded by social isolation and these distinctions in the gravity and depth of poverty are important, particularly when reflecting on the consequences for children and their well-being. A child's economic condition is inextricably linked to their family unit. Therefore, policy investments supporting family economic health by diminishing poverty as an ACE are vital to increasing opportunities for children and the prosperity of our society (Hughes & Tucker, 2018).

Chronic poverty may not be restricted to neighborhoods, families, or individuals that have been under-resourced; on the contrary, chronic poverty flourishes in the larger system that they are entrenched in. Structural dynamic forces and root causes of an inequitable allocation of social resources must be addressed in an intentional manner (Halfon, 2016). Strategic interventions are required in the realm of public policy investments to end child poverty. Lessons can be learned by the English, for instance, development of the Sure Start local programs sponsored by the Blair and Brown governments (Halfon, 2016). The Sure Start local program, an essential approach to eradicate child poverty in a generation, comprises contemporary settlement houses with an array of other community connections and deep investment by the government—$12 billion per year. Favorable changes in child outcomes have been realized. The Sure Start program has components that take after Head Start centers in the US. Since England is approximately one-tenth the size of the US, to pursue comparable efforts the US would need to create 35,000 Sure Start programs, make an endowment of an added $160 billion annually for young children, and ensure that legislative bills are supported and integrated into a cogent cross-agency policy (Halfon, 2016).

Investing in quality early education is another intervention and critical protective factor against the harmful effects of poverty during the earliest years of a child's life as a considerable amount of brain development happens prior to age 5; quality early care experiences are integral to restructuring neural pathways (Hughes & Tucker, 2018). To ensure the preferred lasting effects to combat poverty we recognize that community-wide changes are needed with diminishing risk, improving supports, and creating viable routes to realize personal achievement and community resilience in addition to substantial investment in all people as well as systems upgrades for publicly supported education systems (Halfon, 2016).

If we truly want to realize success for all, a transformative strategy is called for that is informed by complexity science and other comprehensive strategies linked to credible time structures and investment methods. The indisputable deficit of human potential along with the burden of unnecessary malady and disability that harmful inequity is creating can be disregarded only at our own peril (Halfon, 2016).

Homelessness

Homelessness, which frequently stems from consequences of individual traumas (e.g., abuse) and systemic inequalities (e.g., unemployment and discrimination) is an obvious impetus to acknowledge failed policies and social injustice within our society; embedded in this world is widespread inequality, poverty and discrimination (Usman, 2016). Also, trauma and homelessness often coincide and these traumatic incidents indirectly or directly can cause, or even lead to, homelessness (Gulliver & Campney, 2015). Moreover, individuals subjected to homelessness have a greater likelihood of being targets of trauma than individuals who are housed. This takes into account all forms of trauma such as physical and sexual assault.

Youth describe a variety of experiences contributing to their homelessness consisting of social, economic, and environmental influences. In addition, these youths are exposed to numerous, often incessant traumatic stresses, involving victimization. Twenty-five percent of the total youth homeless population has observed domestic violence; 66 percent have been subjected to physical violence (Clervil & DeCandia, 2013). Moreover, by 12 years of age, 83 percent of youth who are homeless have encountered at least one serious violent event (Clervil & DeCandia, 2013). Of note, many youth are subjected to homelessness because of their identity as LGBTQ. They often run away or are banished from their family of origin because of their sexual orientation or gender identity (Forge, Hartinger-Saunders, Wright, & Ruel, 2018). Trauma experienced by homelessness is frequently confounded by earlier incidences of trauma, especially for those who were subjected to involvement with the child welfare system. This group has heightened risk for experiencing sexual trauma, which makes them more inclined to engage in risky sexual behaviors including vulnerability to recruitment into sex trafficking (Forge et al., 2018). What's more, youth who are homeless tend to have limited social assets and low levels of social support. Social support is a major protective factor that defends against adverse experiences and forecasts incidents of homelessness for youth formerly involved in foster care (Forge et al., 2018).

The scale of approaches that can be implemented to remedy homelessness varies. Housing First, a programmatic intervention, focuses on long-term, chronically homeless individuals (Heffernan, Todorow, & Luu, 2015). Its focus is grounded in the belief that individuals require a home prior to being able to attend to addiction and other issues. However, this approach is restrictive since it does not take care of fundamental elements contributing to homelessness or its prevention; it also does not effectively engage the diversity of individuals who are subjected to homelessness (Heffernan et al., 2015). For example, Housing First is put forth as a cure to homelessness for Canada's shortage of reasonably priced housing. Interestingly, Canadian jurisdictions are often employing the Housing First program while also applying public disinvestment from or insufficient recent investment in reasonably priced housing; that is, funding has been slashed to 365,000 low-income families across the country that depend on sponsored housing (Heffernan et al., 2015). In Canada more than 235,000 individuals suffer visible homelessness annually, and no fewer than 1.3 million have been subjected to homelessness or unstable housing over the prior five years (Heffernan et al., 2015). When program interventions are conjectured as remedies to macro-level problems, this can obfuscate regularities of more expansive disinvestment from public infrastructure (Katz, Zerger, & Hwang, 2017). Clearly, it is vital that essential program interventions are not postulated as solutions to challenges such as homelessness, while intentional inaction by the government occurs when macro-level issues are prevalent. Moreover, intervention-related remedies should not obscure the intersecting systems of colonialism, racism, as well as other injustices within our world (Katz et al., 2017).

Taken together, to effectively tackle the causes and restore the influences of homelessness, governmental policies and community supports are necessary. We need more than models that focus on the capability of the individual to attain his or her goals. Intentional widespread efforts must be applied to the community to realize considerable and lasting results; policy and funding linked with national covenants to support affordable housing policy is requisite. Program interventions alone do not have the capacity to resolve leading societal challenges on their own. We must have the political will to adopt a holistic strategy to endorse and carry out policy solutions which promote transformative conditions that greatly increase resources for affordable housing (Katz et al., 2017).

Financial costs of ACEs

ACEs can greatly influence a child's emotional and social well-being as well as physical health however the effects extend considerably beyond these immediate results (Shaffer, Smith, & Ornstein, 2018). Preventing ACEs bears an inherent moral imperative, although other areas require consideration, including its enormous financial burden and to some extent large expenses needed for intervention. An additional element that warrants noting is the immediate and long-term effect on physical wellness, emotional health and functional capabilities. It has been posited that a central reason for limited research in this area is because many researchers retreat at the notion of planning to place an economic appraisal on a youngster's suffering (Shaffer et al., 2018). Nevertheless, growth in evidence, as noted below, elucidates the profound financial cost of ACEs and emphasizes the monetary along with the moral imperative of successful prevention and treatment measures (Gerson & Corwin 2015). Along with substantial individual consequences, the financial costs of early adversity are significant in health care and across other spheres (e.g., child welfare, education, justice, and employment).

Shaffer et al. (2018) report that the lifetime cost of ACEs (2012 dollars) was approximated at $210,012 per child. The general annual economic cost of ACEs in Canada (2017 dollars) was $22.4 billion. When comparing these figures to other chronic health conditions the costs of ACEs has greater than the assessed annual direct and indirect costs related to obesity ($8.4 billion in 2017 dollars) and almost equivalent to tobacco use ($22.25 billion in 2017 dollars) (Shaffer et al., 2018).

According to Bellis et al. (2017), a lone case of non-lethal child abuse is appraised in the US to contribute to life expectancy costs of $10,530 in adult medical needs, in addition to $144,360 in lost productivity. When looking at the effects of financial costs of childhood sexual abuse, the United Kingdom has estimated that the annual expenditures to adult mental health and substance use services was projected to be £178 million (Bellis et al., 2017). In East Asia and the Pacific, it is projected to cost upwards of $194 billion annually (2012 value in US dollars). This is comparable to 2 per cent of the region's gross domestic product (The Commonwealth, 2017).

In Australia, data captured for cases of child abuse in 2012–2013 appraised the overall lifetime economic costs (such as health, welfare, criminal costs, and productivity losses) to be $9.3 billion and the total lifetime non-financial costs (e.g., reduced quality of life and premature mortality) related to incident cases of child abuse to be $17.4 billion (McCarthy et al., 2016).

In San Francisco, a study examining the economic implications of child abuse was conducted specifically in the Bay Area, encompassing the following counties—Alameda, Contra Costa, Marin, Monterey, Napa, San Francisco, San Mateo, Santa Clara, Solano, and Sonoma. The total assessed costs linked with one year of validated cases of child abuse in 2017 in San Francisco was $226.5 million; because of considerable under-reporting of child abuse, the overall financial cost could be up to $6.5 billion (Safe & Sound, 2018). Given contextual factors, San Francisco has community risk-factors that produces greater susceptibility to its residents including the effect of economic volatility and homelessness and relocation of people and immigration. To mitigate risks for ACEs, it is important to strengthen protective factors such as parental resilience, social connections, concrete support in times of need, knowledge of parenting, and social / emotional competence of children (Safe & Sound, 2018). Importantly, while numerous ACEs demonstrate unfavorable mental health concerns along with the taking on of health-harming behaviors, ACEs have a cumulative effect (dose-response relationship); that is, every added ACE experienced boosts risks of adverse health and health-care use (Bellis et al., 2017).

Interventions to help mitigate these costs can be addressed using strategic approaches. First, children's rights need to be elevated universally to transform consequences and mitigate behaviors from ever occurring. Smith (2016) acknowledges that policies need to be transparent and extend voice to the silenced, readdress limited resources to children's services, and hold accountable the state and international community when child-friendly benchmarks are not met (including use of a trauma-informed approach). Children must be seen as individuals with agency and rights to be shielded from injustice, inhumanity, and deprivation— e.g., discrimination, abuse, exploitation, substance abuse, violence. Children have an inherent right to be treated with dignity, respect, and power. Strengthening children's rights requires political and community will and commitment to achieve it (Smith, 2016). Also, earlier in this chapter, we highlighted how poverty and socio-economic conditions with families and children are highly implicated with exposure to abuse or neglect. It is crucial that this link is underscored as a public concern and a matter of unnecessary and preventable social inequality. Universally, data about ACEs must be captured and an evidence base on the extent and nature of the correlation between families' socio-economic conditions and ACEs must be examined as well as linking consequences in adult life and economic costs to test relevant research models. Finally, meaningful anti-poverty policies must be established and interlinked, with policies striving for significantly lower inequities in child health and education, clearly incorporating an emphasis on the relevance for ACEs. Specifically, looking at the influence of anti-poverty policies on ACEs for dissimilar groups of children must be contemplated and addressed, particularly diverse age groups, children functioning with disability, and varied ethnic classification and children residing in mostly deprived communities (Bywaters et al., 2016).

In summary, this chapter highlights the importance of human ecology and community and state level interventions linked with ACEs and how contextual factors cannot be overstated. The context in which an individual grows enfolds them within social forces that can improve or worsen the probability that a person will engage in or adopt health-harming behavior.. The ecosystem of a person's life is exposure to macro-level social-structural forces (e.g., economic, culture, government) and micro-level factors that must be taken into consideration in any attempt to explain how and why a person experiences or participates in aggressive behavior. Taking on a trauma-informed approach is applicable and should be embedded at the policy level, and operated both from an interagency and cross-sectoral standpoint.

PART V

Conclusion

12

MOVING FORWARD

Throughout this book, information has been provided to illustrate both the enduring influence of ACEs on long-term health and well-being as well as realizing that on a macro-level, ACEs are global public health issues. The original ACE Study moves forward our understanding of early life stresses and the health-damaging effects that are implicated in promoting health disparities. There is a vital need for public health endeavors that tackle the social and economic circumstances that are key drivers in health inequalities stemming from ACEs. As well, research on ACEs is needed to move toward evidence to marshal recommended prevention and treatment approaches for individuals along with a wide range of community-based contexts where ACEs assessment, education, and interventions could occur. The science of ACEs is foundational knowledge health professionals must be well-informed about, including health-related policies that unfavorably impinge on families and communities. Health professionals have a responsibility to be knowledgeable of emerging research on ACEs, and this research evidence must be translated into relevant policies that can be executed to advance the needs of vulnerable populations. Taking into account the socio-ecological factors that are implicated in health, research on ACEs, toxic stress, and trauma must provoke a serious look at policies involving poverty, affordable housing, public education, incarceration, human rights, immigration, living wage, as well as access to health and behavioral health services. Health professionals have an ethical imperative to perceive clinical practice within the macro context while making every effort to come to be life-long activists and effective professionals while engaging in work using a social justice lens. It is incumbent on health professionals to vigorously shift from merely thinking about ACEs on an individual level to extend considering mechanisms to address cross-sector collaboration to form healthy communities and upholding policies that encourage resilience and preclude ACEs. Importantly, health professionals have a critical role in not only leading or being integral members on research teams, they are also important as it relates to supporting and advocating for public health measures that prevent and offer early interventions to support health-promoting strategies that strive to produce healthier environments for today's youth, along with making sustainable advances in health at the population level for future generations. In addition to having a strong lens on research, moving forward, health professionals must organize strategies across divisions including education, social, and health to reduce the widespread individual and public ills associated with ACEs.

Research we need

Research is vital to addressing the determinants of ACEs and their effects on health across the lifespan. While evidence presented in earlier chapters suggests that exposure to ACEs arises from adverse social, economic and institutional structures that shape an individual's access to resources and the patterns in their day-to-day, research must occur to scaffold wellness and optimize quality of life especially for populations that are under-resourced and marginalized. ACEs are not arbitrarily dispersed in the population; they are an "endogenous, downstream determinant of health" (Perreira & Gallo, 2017, para. 5). Conducting meaningful research has the capability to decrease the pervasive health burden of ACEs; however it is imperative to distinguish and intervene in the upstream factors that influence exposure to them in the first place. Pointed research agendas incite funders and investigators to target consensus-driven fundamental queries and research methodologies, the outcomes of which can afford evidence to apprise health policies and systems.

To support this initiative, characterizing the central areas for future research can also be promoted by consulting leading organizations in the health professions, particularly those with research and policy committees as well as groups focused on moving toward multi-disciplinary, multi-institutional research collaborations to support prompt dissemination across disciplines to tackle moving forward research on ACEs from a holistic perspective. Given that youth under 18 account for at least 24% of the population in the US, coupled with the understanding of the life course implications of ACEs and their effects on the health of children, the fact that less than 10% of federal expenditures is dedicated to child health and well-being is of huge concern (Fairbrother, Dougherty, Pradhananga, & Simpson, 2017). However, expenditures for child well-being are not responsive to the mounting data regarding the life-course consequences of unfavorable child health (Fairbrother et al., 2017). Research discoveries must be conveyed to policy makers tapping into their frame of reference guiding their ethical mandate which will also necessitate strategic messaging that supports the value framework of policymakers. It will be important for ACE prevention and interventions efforts (individual and multi-level), supported via policy, to examine cost-effectiveness to survey their impact on a national, state, and local level. Wholly appraising ACE effects, both direct and indirect, identifying factors that establish the ability to curtail ACE effects, as well as including a range of protective factors at the individual and community levels, are focal needs when conducting future research.

Social

ACEs are critical social equity and public health issues in the world. It is crucial to push forward reformations, especially prime contributing factors for children and adolescents development of psychological, behavioral, and physiological health concerns—ACEs, which frequently challenge their well-being throughout life (Biglan, Van Ryzin, & Hawkins, 2017). Specifically, the problem of ACEs must be examined within the context of the corrosion of our social communities. Leading areas implicated in this corrosion are poverty, homelessness, drug abuse/overdose, discrimination, coercive family conditions, single parenting and criminal justice (Biglan et al., 2017). Sample domains pertinent to ACEs which can be used to develop relevant research questions are provided. As well, associated implications for these domains are discussed:

(1) Framing child issues so that they grip policy makers, research funders, and leaders

Political positions and ideological viewpoints are integral to swaying policy and research decisions. Matters that are disregarded in the policy realm could also be ignored by researchers. Nevertheless, ongoing gathering of data can propel an assertion to social policy since it would uphold a critical concern–such as ACEs–on an agenda or priority list. Investigations are needed to examine the impact of large-scale multi-level system policies—government, leading health professions organizations, state and community-level— on the best ways to communicate evidence pertaining to ACEs to promote effectiveness of early interventions. Additionally, studying the impact of these policies over the life-course of individuals as well as across generations is warranted. Research that makes recommendations for and assesses the effects of legislation, regulations, and associated actions regarding ACEs helps to move forward a more effective research agenda. Society needs research that correlates with policy to unpack the levers that influence ACE exposure at the structural and institutional levels, and examines how these interrelate with risk and protective elements at the individual, interpersonal and community levels. Outcomes from such research promote a more holistic perspective on how ACEs affect children. Interaction between these levers, risk and protective elements explains how, where, when and why ACEs take place in the life of children. Strong evidence on communication strategies are beneficial at numerous points across the spectrum and in different contexts pertaining to ACEs, to evoke a decisive policy response with evidence of underlying factors that produce ACEs. In some instances, meaningful action-oriented processes may necessitate a moral charge and the will of politicians and others to move forward a profound strategy to dissolve ACEs.

(2) Poverty as a central social influencer of child well-being

Poverty is a leading intractable issue facing our communities and it adversely affects almost every marker of child well-being and affects more than one in five children. Children from birth to 5 years are developmentally most vulnerable to poverty's impacts. Research can guide policy and resources to have a considerable bearing on the economic well-being of children and families. Poverty is a robust element in the accumulation of ACEs and subsequent toxic stress associated with poor outcomes for youth. A child's economic conditions are inextricably linked to those of their families; social policy that encourages family financial health also helps to lessen poverty (Hughes & Tucker, 2018). Research questions that address cross-sector areas and incorporates modeling that takes into account the racialization of social, economic, and institutional structures in society is required. Racial and ethnic differences in the pervasiveness of ACEs manifest the historical and present-day constraints on opportunity and resources, which impinges on every facet of life (Perreira & Gallo, 2017). Thus, prevention and early intervention efforts of ACEs are possible but require intervention at the local, state, and federal levels. Similarly, the development of approaches for reliably detecting ACE-exposed individuals who would benefit from early intervention is warranted. Likewise, research intended to develop and endorse preventative and corrective interventions, especially concerning their long-term impact would be highly regarded. For instance, research can examine the life-course effects of poverty and social factors experienced during childhood and also observe the effects of poverty relief on long-term outcomes (Fairbrother et al., 2017). Research questions that lead to outcomes providing best practice policies and evidence-based programmatic strategies that diminish prevalence and consequences of ACEs and toxic stress are needed. Along with this, examining the return on investment over the life-course of these novel and innovative interventions is warranted (Fairbrother et al., 2017). Moving forward, ACE research (prevention, early intervention and treatment) should be persistent with critically examining practices used to enumerate and codify ACEs that impact children, positioning identification of process and power at the core of research endeavors that are undertaken.

(3) Achieving prosocial family structures that optimize outcomes of children from varied backgrounds

Research must meticulously assess the influence of ACEs on family conditions that directly and indirectly influence youth development. Evaluation research of programs and policies is integral to designate those that demonstrate efficacy and are supportive of families. Designing culturally relevant research for parents that are vulnerable is a high priority to gain insights on the most appropriate resources and environments needed to best equip them to supply safe, stable, nurturing relationships and settings for their children. As an example, policies that bolster family financial status (e.g. allocating livable earnings and compensated family leave) can relieve parental stress, an acknowledged risk factor for ACEs; in addition, it can enable parents to afford resources to sustain their children's fundamental needs in order to thrive.

Investigating best practice approaches to messaging a shared value-based approach concerning youth well-being that also focusses on the outcomes on the family would serve to be invaluable. Furthermore, research protocols are needed to identify and test (1) family and youth-centered approaches to measure and discuss ACEs and (2) requisite self-care, resilience, and relationship skills in a wide-range of settings. Research is also called for to develop and demonstrate models that attend to ACEs and healthy parenting in diverse settings and among low-resourced populations. Also, identifying and executing family-friendly work policies that can be used to decrease ACE exposure is needed. Similarly, exploring the effects of multi-level, action-focused, non-health-related policies on neighborhood and community conditions and their ability to decrease ACEs and promote family social cohesion is required. Policy-level strategies with allocated resources must consider how contextual needs can have significant impact on ACEs by safeguarding the conditions in which families can thrive. This is key to increasing the probability that ACEs will not continue to go on. However, it is vital that we ask the right questions, since these questions are inextricably linked to the outcome of addressing the problem. Another area of significant influence on family cohesion is the deleterious effects of the criminal justice system's overly punitive practices on marginalized and historically racial minority populations. Research that extends data on how incarceration destabilizes family financial well-being and strength will be essential in developing policies urging the justice system to evaluate policies that harm families, and to equitably institute practices among all populations (Biglan et al., 2017).

Intentional and proactive practices are pivotal when research questions are developed and selected, including what interventions are tracked to affect ACEs that impact youth, families, and communities. Family development within environments of adversity offers copious salient research paths from the micro-processes between children and their caretakers to the macro-processes of policies that improve or exacerbate children's exposure to ACEs. ACE data must direct community assets, adopt intersectoral collaboration, and strive to improve an individual's well-being. Examining macro-level factors that impel ACEs must be made visible in order to address this problem, including surveying how universal, economic, and political processes affect the dynamics of ACEs. We need to learn additional information about what is driving ACEs at a population-level along with how that relates to individual-level risks. Consequentially, it is likely that research needed includes ecological and multi-level experiments, accompanied by long-term qualitative and ethnographic exploration. Ultimately, ACE-related data shapes initiatives at the individual, population, and policy levels and inspires culturally-relevant interventions to move forward desired outcomes we wish to realize in society.

Education

Worldwide, school context is frequently a place where children tend to spend the majority of their time compared to other settings external to their home setting. School settings can be places where ACEs are furthered or places that promote well-being and inclusion. Research is a priority that examines educational outcomes of children exposed to ACEs elucidating the intricacies of interdependent relationships between and among people and groups of people as well as cultural resources such as viewpoints of all members of the school community, pertinent resources, and community and society issues that influence education and learning (Berg, Osher, Moroney, & Yoder, 2017). Research on the capacity to deliver a positive school climate with favorable emotional and social development is needed for all students, including those with elevated ACEs, irrespective of culture, race, socioeconomic position, sexual and gender orientation as well as disability status. While the US is lowest among 32 high-resource countries in social and emotional learning in schools, cross-sectional groups (e. g., policymakers, researchers, and health professionals) in the US and internationally are progressively indicating the desire for positive school conditions and the promotion of social and emotional skills in schools (Biglan et al., 2017). Also, the National Survey of Children's Health reports that less than 48% of school-age children in the US meet fundamental conditions to flourish. Therefore, action-oriented research strategies tackling micro- and macro-level factors to mitigate ACEs and strengthen healthy schools must be embarked on to effectively support populations with limited political influence due to structures that embrace inequities in well-being. Consequently, research is needed that examines provisions for cross-sector collaboration to stimulate action and deal with structural inequalities. Research should be adopted that identifies gaps related to service quality, professional capacity and competence, professional mechanisms for upholding positive early education years of transitions for children exposed to ACEs. Moreover, evaluating efforts to broaden knowledge about applications of trauma-informed practices across spectrums of the educational realm would further extend understanding of its effect for those impacted by ACEs. Also, identifying how trauma-exposed students in a trauma-informed school setting thrive in their school site compared to those in traditional school sites with similar backgrounds can serve to be beneficial. As ACEs research evolves that addresses many of these challenges, it would be helpful to incorporate integrative multi-level, transdisciplinary systems and professionals given that inequities in education and exposure to ACEs have their origins in the structure of society and manifest the disparate life opportunities.

Health

The original ACE Study occurred two decades ago and its findings have resulted in ACEs being recognized as a public health crisis necessitating a multidimensional research response.

Research has supported association of ACEs with increased risk of physical and behavioral health difficulties; however no causal links have been established between ACEs and effects on the brain and health outcomes. Research that ascertains the extent of the causality between ACEs and deleterious outcomes late in life, and the processes through which this takes place is needed (UK Parliament, 2018). There are chasms in the evidence-base regarding ACEs and later outcomes, to some extent, from limited capability to connect longitudinal survey data to governmental or insurance documents to afford a more comprehensive picture of individuals' life stories and to gain improved insight on how various facets of individuals' lives interrelate (UK Parliament, 2018). Deeper understanding is vital on how implications from ACE exposure enters the body, modifying lasting pathogenesis which predisposes an individual to undesirable health outcomes. As Naguib Mahvouz states, "nothing records the effects of a sad life as graphically as the human body." Literature also indicates the significance of the timing of ACEs, especially when health development occurs during sensitive periods (Halfon, Larson, Son, Lu, & Bethell, 2017). Importantly, cross-sectional research is common. However, this mitigates opportunities to gain important information; research is necessary that can pinpoint the timing, duration, or interactions of precise exposures to ACEs that impacts health outcomes. This is critical as timing is important along with context and the presence of counteracting protective factors that can moderate the role that ACEs have on particular health outcomes (Halfon et al., 2017). Timing is key, as it relates to the age of the child as well as the intensity and duration of exposure to an ACE or ACEs. Likewise, it is important to accurately know if and how ACEs are transgenerationally transmitted and understanding the mechanisms by which this occurs (Halfon et al., 2017). When examining implications of ACEs, it would be helpful to elucidate how biological sensitivity to context arises and is altered by different signals from both gradual and hastily changing environmental effects.

Of great importance is translating ACE Study findings to deter adversity in childhood and research that promotes early intervention, prevention, and positive health. This is the undergirding of the science of ACEs (exploration of ACE characteristics, evolution, prevalence, and effects) and the knowledge development on resilience and thriving (see Center on Developing Child, Harvard University). The premise of early interventions is that intervening earlier is advantageous. The prevention of ACEs is warranted merely by diminishing children's exposure to ACEs. Evidence focused on ACEs, resilience factors, and undesirable outcomes in later life implies that resources expended on tackling matters including physical and mental health or criminal acts would be better suited to address more immediate opportunities for intervention. Evaluation of early interventions should be operationalized in real-world settings to examine the effect on actual communities where delivery occurs. Research that can discern delivery of high-quality services to individuals, specifically interventions with the applicable characteristics of quality, supplied at the right time, measuring desired transformation related to when it works, for whom, how the interventions work as well as how outcomes can be enhanced, are pertinent areas of investigation (UK Parliament, 2018). Moving forward, to address ACEs and promote healing and positive health, Halfon et al. (2017) argues that we must institute a "purposeful research, policy analysis, technical assistance, and funding-assistance infrastructure that enables innovation and real-time learning, improvement, and implementation" (¶ 10).

Research involving those in the health professions who work with individuals exposed to ACEs is also pivotal. For example, Balistreri's (2015) research on delivery of healthcare brings awareness to the value of a medical home model of care on children's well-being. Specifically, this model of care offers continuous and comprehensive care in the early to late stages of life, and is considered a vital tool to move forward the development of systems to care for children, especially those confronting difficulties related to a scarcity of economic means. Given the exposure to ACEs and associated stress that likely comes with them, children who have a medical home available to them tend to have greater levels of well-being comparable to similar children lacking this type of care (Balistreri, 2015). Moving forward, research would be invaluable to examine the characteristics embodied by medical homes that deliver protective mechanisms for those who have experienced ACEs (Balistreri, 2015). Future research should also critically examine what types of health-related interactions benefit trauma survivors to effectively modify health behavior (Raja, Hasnain, Hoersch, Goe-Yin, & Rajagopalan, 2015), along with comparing care delivered among health providers who have a fundamental understanding of the health implications of ACEs, compared to those who lack this knowledge. Research is also needed that distinguishes mechanisms that influence educated providers to engage ACE exposed individuals in preventive care and whether this engagement prevents or decreases undesirable coping behaviors (Raja et al., 2015). Inquiries that result in findings that demonstrate evidenced-based research regarding methods that are useful to engage and support individuals who were subjected to ACEs during their childhood would move forward practices to be able to ask about ACEs self-assuredly and reply appropriately. Furthermore, other research questions and ideas to consider include:

- Assessing the relationship between knowledge of ACEs and trauma-informed practices and diverse fields of health professions.
- Distinguishing how providers use trauma-informed practices across different settings including the frequency of these practices.
- Examining barriers perceived by providers to applying trauma-informed practices.
- What are health care providers' own trauma histories and what are the implications from this on addressing ACEs and trauma among individuals they care for?

As a community, moving forward from adverse experiences, such as ACEs and trauma, is attained through fostering resilience, embedded in both the physiology of adaptation and the incidents we subject our children to. Research on the nature of resilience and ACEs is integral especially with investigating the paths of moderation and prevention of ACEs for adults and children. Investigations are needed to assess what renders some children and adolescents resilient when exposed to ACEs, and in which situations families disrupt the progression of the intergenerational transmission of adversity. Harvard University's National Scientific Council on the Developing Child endorses the concept that resilience is a tool and, when taken on by children early in life, develops into normative behavior as they move into adulthood. Conducting research to test resilience-based methods to ACEs can provide effective intervention approaches at the individual, family, organization, or community level (Make It So, 2016). In moving forward with development of resilience approaches and processes, it is vital to observe the humanitarian priority of Do No Harm (Wessells, 2015). Therefore, a resilience approach must not divert attention from promoting justice and equity as well as associated issues of chronic poverty, exclusion, and structural violence which are foundational sources for risk accumulation that harms the lives of considerable numbers of children globally (Wessells, 2015). Neither should a resilience focus conceal the distress and needs of children that require clinical supports. We must hold up resilience and attend conscientiously to our ethical obligations to seek strategies that support children in times of highest need (Wessells, 2015).

In summary, meaningful research which considers micro- to macro-level issues must be promoted, including conscientiously studying the influence of each segment of society on family and educational conditions that are integrally influential on child development. While not exhaustive, we discussed some pertinent areas that would be invaluable to investigate. Utilizing historic and evolving research on ACEs and trauma allows investigators to leverage opportunities for well-being and maintain hope for prevention, alleviation, and healing of individual, intergenerational, and community trauma related to ACE exposure. Also, research must not occur in silos; relevant findings must be implemented via policy provisions, with associated resources to carry them out in order to enhance children's chances of developing successfully, promote healthy families and wholesome communities.

The society we could have

ACEs are preventable and every person has a part to play; embracing comprehensive solutions is at the core. The outlook of any society hinges on its ability to promote the healthy development of the next generation—all of our children. If we authentically want progressive change regarding ACEs and their impact on society, we need to be prepared to speak about them. We are not equipped to expose something that is not being looked for or made visible. Therefore, as individuals in society elevate their consciousness of the pandemic existence of ACEs, we must cultivate practices of inquiry that will allow individuals across the lifespan to communicate their story and reveal incidents which may be transpiring or may have transpired. As Maya Angelou stated *"There is no greater agony than bearing an untold story inside you"* (Guardian, 2014, p. 1). Our social climate must enable us all to think about unthinkable behaviors that individuals may be confronted with, particularly children. Our society has a moral obligation to advocate on behalf of children and protect them from harm. We must use the science developed that provides evidence-based strategies and those that offer best practices and continue to be informed by useful future developments. ACE prevention and intervention should not be a controversial issue; children lack control over their exposure to adverse experiences. We must urgently encourage and direct clinicians, researchers, and policymakers to implement practices, sponsor and fund legislation to inhibit child trauma exposure, and to expeditiously intercept the effects if protection is not successful.

ACEs are strongly interconnected with a wide-ranging gamut of social conditions within society. To move towards having a more desirable society, we have to minimize isolation from one another, since solutions to ACEs require comprehensive and interconnected strategies. It would be prudent to identify natural partners whose efforts have a desirable effect on ACE prevention even when their motivation or appeal may not be exclusively about ACE prevention. Collectively, cities and members in their social environment must reconsider what comprises meaningful ACE prevention strategies. Fostering prosocial ideals and goals that scaffold efforts to apply agendas, programs, procedures, and cultural practices is integral for society to enhance the number of families, educational settings, and communities that cultivate the well-being of each individual (Biglan et al., 2017). The effect of ACEs on human well-being is strong enough to make paramount the imperative to advance society's prevention of ACEs. Development of prevailing health care and human services systems in society is needed to move forward broad, effective execution of interventions. Ensuring a foundation to realize a society where virtually all youth reach adulthood with the necessary skills, ideals, and health practices is essential to promoting productive lives (Biglan et al., 2017).

If, as a society, we would simply realize that trying to repair the human body after we allow it to be broken is always more detrimental and costly compared to not shattering it in the beginning, as Bloom (2016) states, "we could all live in a land of plenty" (p. 394). This demands a move from the traditional stated ideal of individualism to caring for the collective. Moreover, it requires refocusing; specifically, thinking of a triumphant system as short-term profitability along with the sole value of matter being money. As a society, we have a moral charge to act with the knowledge that ACEs and adversity brought about in the world at present are preventable (Bloom, 2016). Surely we have the ability, and with determination we can infuse hope, promise and the will to eliminate ACEs by investing in humanity to promote equity in health, create a future worth surviving, and a society aspiring for justice.

"The way you help to heal the world [from ACEs] is you start with your own community."

(Mother Teresa, Goodreads, 2019, p. 1)

APPENDIX 1: INTEGRATING ACE EDUCATION INTO THE CURRICULUM OF HEALTH PROFESSIONALS

It is posited that trauma recovery and healing begins with education; therefore it is imperative that health care professionals take on the ethical responsibility to deliver that education to those they serve. Within this addendum, we will examine examples of the current status of inclusion of science on adverse childhood experiences (ACEs) and trauma-informed information in the educational curricula for health care professionals at the baccalaureate, masters and doctoral levels. Additionally, recommendations for faculty regarding the necessity for new models that reflect the need for intentional integration of the current knowledge about the effects of chronic stress, adversity, and trauma will be offered.

Our guiding principle for the recommendations proffered in this appendix follows the thinking of Richard Buckminster Fuller (Buckminster Fuller Institute, n.d.), "You never change things by fighting the existing reality. To change something, build a new model that makes the existing model obsolete" (¶ 1).

There are more than two decades of professional research, scholarly papers, and books filled with findings and information on trauma and its effects (Anda et al., 2006; Flaherty et al., 2013). The original ACE study is more than two decades old, yet the curricula in health care education are often devoid of any but cursory information on the effects of adversity, chronic stress, and trauma on populations of people that health care professionals care for. How then will these professionals recognize, assess, teach, and offer effective help? As Kathleen Wheeler (2018), noted nursing expert, stated, "It is time for all nurses to lift their professional blinders and begin a new era of care for those populations most vulnerable to the causes and consequences of trauma" (p. 20). These blinders, common to all health care professionals, and likely held in place as much by individual and societal needs for denial and dissociation of human vulnerability and historical oppression as lack of information, require removal if health care professionals are to be prepared for practice.

There are few students in fields of study that are trauma-related who receive formal training in psychological trauma or the impact of ACEs on individuals, families and communities. Those students who have exposure are the fortunate few who have professors and clinical mentors knowledgeable in the area of trauma training (Miller, Conrad, Brady, Moffitt, & Bay, 2004). Rather, the majority of professionals are left to pick their way through offerings in continuing education programs, professional conferences and books and journal articles pertaining to trauma. Courtois and Gold (2009) state, "Obviously, this alternative is a relatively haphazard one in that it does not reflect the planning, structure, comprehensiveness, and supervised practice that are the hallmarks of an organized professional training program, especially where direct services are involved" (p. 4).

The authors propose that, in order to "ace" health care professionals' education and prepare those professionals for practice, didactic education, and clinical training must incorporate and integrate in-depth information on chronic adversity, stress, trauma, and its effects. The ACE study provides the scientific basis for the dissolution of the mind/body dichotomy, making the integration of the effects of stress on individuals key to developing competency for practice. Additionally, burgeoning knowledge cited in this book's chapters regarding epigenetics and brain science serves as a call for action to mandate integration of these elements in health care education. There are thought and action leaders who have begun to address the critical need for inclusion of ACEs science and a trauma-informed focus with the goal of educating those students and health professionals. For example, the Philadelphia ACE Task Force (PATF), a network of professionals driven by a desire to improve health through the application of ACEs information, developed a work group to examine the state of incorporation of this knowledge into curricula. The work group conducted an environmental scan of ACE and trauma-informed courses comprising all levels of education programs (Felter & Ayers, 2016). The group found that universities and colleges in the Northeast and the West regions of the United States contained the largest concentrations of trauma education components. Additionally, the work group scanned for ACEs and trauma-based program offerings according to field of study revealing that Social Work topped the list, followed by Psychology and Counseling/Therapy fields. Medicine ranked fourth with eight offerings and Nursing was seventh on the list with a paltry three offerings of trauma-based information (Felter & Ayers, 2016). In the report, *Incorporating Trauma Informed Practice and ACEs into Professional Curricula Toolkit* (Felter & Ayers, 2016), the work group also scanned for levels of educational opportunities according to type and found that the majority of offerings were in the form of courses, research projects and certificate programs with many fewer educational curricula proffering programs, tracks, and concentrations with a trauma-informed focus. These findings, along with a database of undergraduate and graduate education in trauma psychology published earlier by the Education and Training Committee of the American Psychological Association, point to the deep gap in ACEs and trauma education and training in college and university programs.

Health care professionals are a diverse group but they share in common the care of human beings of varying ages and backgrounds who are in need of intervention to assist them with their health and well-being. The traditional medical model that underlies much of health care education and practice frames care around labeling or diagnosing; however, the lens of trauma-informed education and practice looks for the context, that is what is behind and surrounding the diagnosis. This context is filled with complexity, including person intrinsic factors as well as extrinsic factors such as the surrounding physical, familial, community, and cultural environments. Additionally, the power structures that are inherent to health care include the health care professionals' actual capacity to label and diagnose. Furthermore, the structural understanding of health that includes issues of structural violence and structural vulnerability are of primary importance to the health care professional's education if they are to more fully understand the breadth of effects of trauma and adversity (Thompson-Lastad et al., 2017). These factors, which are often overlooked and typically not integrated into health care education, exert a profound influence on the content and process of care and must be accounted for.

Acing education requires a shift to a unifying paradigm that teaches the necessary knowledge about the effects of chronic stress, adversity and trauma across the life span and couples this knowledge with the development of skills for assessment, prevention, intervention and evaluation. As critical to this paradigm shift is an analysis of the attitudes and assumptions the health care professional brings to practice. Courtois and Gold (2009) recommend the inclusion of trauma-related information and topics from the undergraduate level onward. The emerging literature pertaining to incorporation of the teaching of trauma in health care student curricula includes Matta, Woodward-Kron, Petty, and Salzber (2016) who offer six concepts for consideration:

> communication skills; knowledge of the health effects of trauma and abuse; knowledge about the effects of trauma and abuse disclosures on doctors and other health professions; specific knowledge relevant to different medical specialties and settings; teaching formats and methods; and the need for a staged, incremental, integrated program, structured to achieve continuity between undergraduate, prevocational and specialist phases.
>
> *(p. 248)*

As the effects of chronic adversity and toxic levels of stress are more fully recognized as deleterious factors in human development, their ubiquitous presence must be recognized and incorporated into a fuller understanding of what constitutes health, illness, and human resilience and must be included as basic and integrated knowledge in the education of health care professionals. The infusion of ACEs correlates and health outcomes into health care education broadens understanding of the multiple factors influencing health, improves accuracy of diagnosis, and guides the interventions of the provider in the direction of effective partnership, with those served thus promoting better chances for positive outcomes. Models of curricula that intentionally integrate cultural and structural competencies throughout may serve as templates for this endeavor.

Undergraduate education

There are a plethora of opportunities for the inclusion of ACEs science and information on stress/chronic adversity and trauma to be integrated into core courses taught in undergraduate programs. The information presented in the book chapters on early brain development and epigenetics calls for the incorporation of this knowledge in foundational science courses such as microbiology and anatomy and physiology. More advanced science courses such as applied cellular biology and genetics should explicate the most current knowledge on effects of stress and trauma. Equally essential is the inclusion of these areas in courses in the health professions such as developmental psychology, health assessment throughout the life span, basics of public health, addictions theory, and courses that seek to build the knowledge base about the social, cultural and economic determinants of health. In addition, courses in health care policy and leadership are comprehensive only if they assure inclusion of the profound influences and implications of social determinants of health to the formulation of equitable health care reform.

An informal survey of educational institutions produced a variety of outcomes demonstrating inclusion of ACE information across associates, baccalaureate, masters and doctoral levels of education. For example, Drexel University offers an undergraduate course in the College of Nursing and Health Professions titled *Trauma-Informed Care* that introduces students to the psychophysiology of complex trauma and includes a requirement that students review and present case studies of children and adolescents who have experienced effects of trauma (Drexel University, 2018). In addition, at the Community College of Philadelphia, a professor of nursing introduced a practice of having nursing students in an associate degree of nursing program take the ACE assessment and derive their own ACE score in an effort to increase awareness of the ways in which adversity operated in the lives of the students (L. Tavolaro-Ryley, personal communication, April 25, 2018). This professor also organized training for all nursing faculty on trauma-informed care as well as requiring that every student take a one-hour trauma-informed principles class. She has noted that, as a result of this training, faculty are including ACEs information in adult health classes presenting ACEs as risk factors for entities such as chronic obstructive pulmonary disease (L. Tavolaro-Ryley, personal communication, April 25, 2018). The practice of requesting students derive their own ACE score, although undoubtedly a self-awareness building exercise, brings to the forefront the need for understanding of the effects of introducing trauma related materials to students. Girouard and Bailey (2017) emphasize the need to assure the health and well-being of students in the health profession via education about their own exposure to ACEs and traumatic incidents. Additionally, courses that explore the nature of trauma as well as symptoms, reactions, and stories related to trauma may produce stressful and, at times, overwhelmed responses in the students exposed to them and may engender a secondary traumatic stress response. Cless and Nelson-Goff (2017) advocate for a model of trauma-informed teaching to be implemented in the classroom in order to mitigate against the development of secondary traumatic stress. They emphasize the risk of emotional reactivity to learning about traumatic material, whether the student has a past experience of trauma potentially putting them at higher risk, or is simply exposed to traumatic material in the course work that may generate reactions. Students need to be equipped with affect regulation skills as well as self-care practices in order to manage more effectively. In addition, the authors recommend the inclusion of reflective supervision practices to help ensure the well-being of the students. We will elaborate on faculty needs and responsibilities in another section.

Graduate education

On the graduate level, inclusion of ACEs science is essential in courses such as advanced health assessment and diagnostic reasoning, neurobiology of trauma, historical and socio-cultural influences on health and evaluation/research of health outcomes. Those students educated at a graduate level are likely to function in health care practices, educational institutions and research facilities. They will be responsible for assessment, design, and delivery of care; therefore, essential in their education is skill development in principles and methods of delivering basic trauma education to patients in culturally sensitive and structurally aware ways. Additionally, health care education programs in general need to integrate information in knowledge areas such as epigenetics in order to define mechanisms by which trauma and stress responses can be transmitted generationally. Those educated at a graduate level will lead research and education initiatives as well as effect policy regarding the structural components of the health care system requiring intervention. Therefore, it is critical that education at this level include in-depth examination of ACE science and its implications for development of prevention initiatives as well as future curricula that must integrate this information and develop best practices.

In the informal survey of graduate education conducted, the authors identified a master's degree program in the Department of Counseling and Family Therapy at Drexel University in Philadelphia that requires several courses in trauma-informed care. These courses include content on historical and sociopolitical underpinnings, neurobiology and neuroplasticity and the effect trauma has on brain development, complex trauma, and its impact on multiple life domains, reviews of cultural considerations' impact and response to trauma, the professional imperative to assess without re-traumatizing people, stages of trauma recovery and treatment modalities as well as community healing opportunities. Another program course covers trauma and families and notes learning goals that include utilizing environmental, psychological, biological, social, and spiritual determinants of health in trauma assessment and practice (L. Schmidt, personal communication, April 16, 2018). At Jefferson University in Philadelphia, Pennsylvania, a graduate-level program that prepares students with a master's in community and trauma counseling fully integrates ACEs science and trauma-centered principles and practices in its curriculum with the majority of some twenty courses including information on trauma-informed principles and practices (J. Felter, personal communication, February 23, 2018). Widener University in Chester, Pennsylvania offers an on-line Master in Social Work degree that focuses on trauma as a root cause of illness and graduates social workers who want to function in a clinical role (Widener University, 2018).

In an effort to assess implications of incorporation of ACE science principles in education, Strait and Bolman (2017) performed a study of 967 students from 9 health profession programs who received curriculum focused on ACEs and trauma-informed care in an inter-professional education course that requested students assess their own ACE score. The outcome data supported their hypothesis that students who voluntarily obtained their own scores were significantly more likely to understand the scientific and clinical findings of the ACEs study and trauma-informed care. The researchers suggest that a follow-up longitudinal study throughout the careers of these participants might illustrate how their approach to patient care may differ along lines of better development of understanding and trust with those under their care. Studies have shown that many who enter the health care professions do so with their own histories of stress, traumatic experiences and significant ACE scores (Maunder, Peladeau, Savage, & Lancee, 2010; Freeman, 2017). In a study conducted by Freeman at the University of Calgary, 112 family medicine residents did not screen their patients for ACEs at high rates; however, residents with a personal history of ACEs were more likely to screen. Those residents more likely to screen were discovered to have a prevalence rate of ACEs comparable to the overall population (Freeman, 2017). Additionally, as mentioned previously, health care professions regularly expose practitioners to the stressful and traumatic incidents in their patients' lives, requiring knowledge of the effects on the practitioner as well as the need for the practice of self-care strategies to minimize negative outcomes for the practitioner and patient. Essential as well, given this data, is the inclusion of trauma education information related to the building of provider resilience in order to support them throughout their professional lives.

The American Psychological Association (2015) has published guidelines on trauma competencies for education that can serve as a model for curriculum which the authors believe will equip the health care professional for practicing from a trauma-informed perspective. The following is derived from the set of the American Psychological Association competencies that are defined as inclusive of knowledge, skills, and attitudes. Crosscutting Competencies are those that are foundational to all and demonstrate:

- The ability to appreciate and understand the impact of trauma and ACEs on health outcomes, the contribution of trauma to increasing health disparities, and the impact of trauma-informed care as a critical component of care for people who are survivors of trauma.
- Understanding about trauma reactions and tailor interventions and assessments in ways that honor and account for individual, cultural, community, and organizational diversity.
- Understanding of how trauma and ACEs impact the individual, the family, the community and the organizations' sense of safety and trust and how to respond in a professional manner to promote safety and trust.
- Understanding and ability to tailor assessment and interventions to account for developmental lifespan factors at the time and duration of ACEs or trauma as well as at the point of professional contact.
- The ability to understand, assess, and tailor interventions and assessments that address the complexities of ACEs and trauma exposure as well as any resultant long and short-term effects such as comorbidities.
- The ability to appropriately appreciate, assess, and incorporate the trauma and ACEs survivors' strengths, resilience and potential for growth.
- The ability to recognize practitioners' capacity for self-reflection and tolerance for intense content; ethical responsibility for self-care and self-awareness of how one's own history, values, and vulnerabilities impact care.
- The ability to understand the value and purpose of the various professional, paraprofessional, and lay responders in the work in order to work collaboratively across systems to enhance positive outcomes..

These competencies represent a fairly comprehensive acknowledgement of patient-related needs and rights, as well as representing many of the health care student's areas of knowledge necessary for competent practice.

Turning the focus to the macro-level of intervention, the Child Poverty Education Subcommittee of the Academic Pediatric Association Task Force on Child Poverty described the development of a curriculum on child poverty for inclusion in undergraduate and graduate medical education settings (Chamberlain et al., 2016). Notably, as ACEs studies evolved to include broader criteria related to the social determinants of health, poverty and its ramifications became an important focus. Key elements of the aforementioned curriculum include the following domains of competence:

- Patient Care: for example, the relevance of gathering essential information on the behavioral, psychosocial, environmental and family unit correlates pertinent to care.
- Interpersonal and Communication Skills: for example, the importance of developing skills to communicate across a broad range of socioeconomic and cultural backgrounds.
- Systems-Based Practice: for example, incorporating considerations of cost awareness and risk-benefit analysis in patient and/or population-based care as well as advocating for optimal patient care systems.
- Professionalism: for example, the development of humanism, compassion, integrity and respect for others as well as a sense of accountability to patients.

(Chamberlain et al., 2016, p. S156)

Garner (2016) asserts that models of health change as the basic sciences advance therefore the models that are used to frame research, teach the upcoming generation of providers and inform public policy must also evolve. The biomedical model of old framed health as the absence of disease and eventually gave way to include the biopsychosocial model with its understanding of health as the product of multiple factors. Scientific advances in developmental neuroscience and epigenetics, for example, have driven the formation of a model of health that acknowledges and integrates the ecological and developmental origins of both illness and wellness (Garner, 2016). Importantly, health care education must keep pace with these developments, which, at the present, include viewing ACEs through the social/ecological lens and integrating structural elements that lend crucial insights to the understanding of health and illness. It is now insufficient to focus on cultural competency which emphasizes the need to identify practitioner awareness of bias and improve professionals' understanding and communication when engaging in the delivery of health care; rather, there is an imperative to comprehend how the economic, political and social conditions bring about health disparities and impede efforts to prevent, treat and restore health to people. This shift, which the authors endorse, includes the following skills that constitute key areas of structural competency enumerated by Metzl and Hansen (2014):

- Recognizing the structures that shape clinical interactions, such as social conditions and institutional policies that shape patient presentation.
- Developing an extra-clinical language of structure that incorporates more complex understanding of social structures and their impact on health.
- Rearticulating cultural formulations in structural terms by accounting for neighborhood and institutional factors.
- Observing and enacting structural interventions through community-based projects that address patient needs.
- Developing structural humility through community and interdisciplinary collaborations alongside the reality that systemic change often requires long-term commitment resulting in progressive change.

Certificate programs

An informal survey of the educational offerings on trauma in the form of certificate programs produced a plethora of options for continuing education in the trauma field. There are numerous on-line trauma trainings and some are offered free of charge. These certificate programs offer learning opportunities in child mental health, information designed to provide resources for the creation of trauma-sensitive schools, as well as web-based courses on specific trauma-focused skill acquisition. The School of Social Work at the University of Buffalo offers several online trauma-informed certificate programs including a trauma-informed clinical foundation program, a certificate program focused on trauma-informed care and counseling as well as a program which is designed to help organizations create trauma-informed cultures (University of Buffalo, 2018). The Traumatology Institute based in Canada offers certificates of completion to those who are pursuing or have completed a Master's degree. This organization's certificate programs include courses for those seeking further training as clinical traumatologists, community and workplace traumatologists, early intervention traumatologists and those interested in learning about trauma-informed practices for use in schools and justice systems. One of the certificate programs includes an emphasis on caregiver stress using a Compassion Fatigue recovery model (Traumatology Institute, 2012). The International Society for Traumatic Stress Studies offers multiple on-line advanced training certificate programs and awards certificates of completion for their programs. The organization clarifies that completion of programs does not constitute certification in trauma (International Society for Traumatic Stress Studies, 2018). Some certificate programs offer certification in a specific area such as Trauma-Focused Cognitive Behavioral Therapy which require prerequisites in terms of degree and licensure in addition to coursework, supervision and practice cases and a passing grade on a knowledge-based test (Therapist Certification Program, 2018). These programs, although providing value to the practitioner are viewed by the authors as adjunct to an integrated, comprehensive and structured curricula based on ACE science and trauma-informed principles and practices.

Clinical training

As students begin their foray into clinical training and engage in clinical rotations, it is essential that didactic information acquired be translated and embedded in practice if we are to turn out clinically competent and trauma-informed practitioners. Trauma-informed clinical practice expertise is relevant in all clinical specialties with variants depending on the setting. Matta et al. (2016) caution that the realities of the work setting, for example, those settings that lack privacy, should not be an excuse for consistently avoiding trauma-informed practices. In clinical training, communication skills, particularly ones that afford opportunities to address trauma-specific areas require emphasis. Clinical simulations can provide occasions to practice these communication skills and may reveal discomfort levels regarding assessing and responding to trauma-related disclosures while providing opportunities to process this discomfort. Trauma-informed clinical education must include and support the practice of screening for stress, adversity, and trauma as well as the factors that allow practitioners to offer guidance and referral for assistance for trauma-related issues. Girouard and Bailey (2017) emphasize the need for nurses to be able to engage in thoughtful discussions about trauma in order to destigmatize the experiences and support patients. Clinical educators must themselves be informed as to the science of ACEs as well as the implications of these experiences for health over the life course in order to guide budding practitioners and to effectively incorporate this knowledge base in clinical training. Additionally, clinical educators will best serve their students by including information on the need for competency in the structural factors impacting the delivery of care.

Faculty preparation

In order for health care educational curricula to be effectively trauma-informed, faculty members must be adequately prepared to deliver such an educational effort. In a resource search for information pertaining to faculty preparation, little was found that addressed the imperative to have a trauma-informed faculty that is well versed in ACEs science and the social and structural determinants of health. In the authors' experience, undergraduate and graduate faculty have frequently called upon practitioners in the trauma-informed fields of practice to deliver guest lectures on these topics. Most certainly the time is overdue for faculty to be prepared to understand and integrate this information throughout both undergraduate and graduate curricula. Additionally, Girouard and Bailey (2017) state "interprofessional research that assesses providers' knowledge, skills and attitudes about ACEs would be helpful to identify areas for education and support to include in preprofessional and professional education" (p. S17). In addition to research on best practices for inclusion of trauma-informed information in the curricula of health care education, the authors also advocate that licensure and certification exams incorporate questions focused on these areas of expertise. This will insure that all levels of educational preparation of health care professionals incorporate this vital information.

Faculty who teach about ACEs science and trauma-informed principles and practices need to accept the ethical responsibility for not only teaching about trauma but teaching in a trauma-informed manner as well. That is, the teaching process should be informed by and consistent with the content being taught or, in other words, faculty should practice what they preach. Students seeking to be educated in the many fields of health care enter their educational experience with their own life histories. As noted earlier in this addendum, many bring their personal histories of adversity, trauma and stress with them. "Trauma confronts schools with a serious dilemma: how to balance their primary mission of education with the reality that many students need help in dealing with traumatic stress to attend regularly and engage in the learning process" (Ko et al., 2008, p. 398). This reality must be factored into the faculty members' practices within the classroom setting and include the need for creation of trauma-sensitive classrooms as well as the imperative that faculty be informed as to how to respond to students whose classroom experiences expose them to potential triggers that may retraumatize them, (i.e., reactivate trauma-related symptoms via exposure to material that is reminiscent of earlier traumatic events). Additionally, faculty need to be aware that health care students are at risk for vicarious traumatization experiences as a result of hearing about human beings' experiences of trauma and adversity. Faculty need to be prepared to create safety within classrooms and practice settings and to inform students of the potential risk to their emotional well-being that information about the traumatic experiences of others may engender. The International Stress Society's Best Practice Parameters include information for those who teach or conduct trainings that emphasize 1) preparing the learners when case examples could trigger members' trauma reactions in predictable ways, 2) communicating to students the potential impact of trauma work (vicarious, secondary or indirect traumatization) and the duty to self-care and 3) not to require students to participate in individual or group experiential training exercises that encourage self-disclosure about personal histories without first providing informed consent with a genuine option to decline participation (International Society for Traumatic Stress Studies, 2000).

Creating emotionally as well as physically safe learning environments needs to be akin to using principles of universal precautions known to many faculty teaching within health care fields. Faculty cannot be expected to know the trauma histories of the individual students in their classrooms, however, certain principles can be employed that create learning environments favorable to comprehending trauma-informed material while holding to an essential tenet of health care that is, first do no harm. Carello and Butler (2015) promote the development of faculty awareness of specific domains in order to create safety in the classroom. Those domains are the individual characteristics of students, the content and context of what is taught, the requirements of assignments, aspects of both instructor and student behavior and interaction, characteristics of the classroom setting itself, and instruction on the practice of self-care. Cless and Nelson-Goff (2017) advocate for making the course structure and content clear and for assuring that the professor be seen as a resource and a safe person within the instructional environment.

An important aspect of the concept of using universal emotional precautions in the educational curricula related to trauma is the need for instruction on emotional regulation and self-care skills. Faculty can introduce the concept of caring for the health care provider via stressing the importance of self-regulation. There are many resources available for skills training in this area, however of primary importance is the attitude of the faculty, which should include normalizing the need for self-regulation for the student, exposed to disturbing and painful material. Concepts that should be intentionally included within trauma-informed curricula must include topics such as vicarious trauma and the risk and protective factors involved. Also critical is the ethical practice of faculty modeling self-regulatory behaviors. Essential to assisting students with self-care is the introduction and discussion of setting healthy boundaries on student disclosure of their own trauma backgrounds in the educational setting. These boundaries serve as an important protective factor for the student and faculty alike. Faculty must also be well informed as to the available resources such as a student-counseling center within the educational institution for those students who may need to make use of such services.

In conclusion, although the areas for integration of ACEs science and trauma-informed knowledge in curricula and clinical rotations may appear daunting, the goal is to widen the understanding of the impact of stress and adversity on the health and well-being of individuals, families, communities and societies and to equip health care professionals with functioning tools for integrating this knowledge into future practice. This is proving to be a slow, yet worthwhile process, with implications that hold the potential promise to improve the health of individuals, families and communities for the generations to come. As this essential information is integrated, the hope is that the health care professional's lens will deepen and permanently widen, resulting in the production of knowledgeable and empathic health care professionals capable of developing innovative and evolving models of health, and delivering informed and compassionate trauma-informed care.

REFERENCES

Abaek, A., Kinn, L., & Milde, A. (2017). Walking children through a minefield: How professionals experience exploring adverse childhood experiences. *Qualitative Health Research*, 28(2), 231–244.

Abuleil, D. (2017). *Understanding the mechanisms underlying brain plasticity in adult humans*. Waterloo, ON: University of Waterloo. Retrieved from https://uwspace.uwaterloo.ca/bitstream/handle/10012/12429/Abuleil_Dania.pdf?sequence=1&isAllowed=y

Adav, S. S., Subbaiaih, R. S., Kerk, S. K., Lee, A. Y., Lai, H. Y., Ng, K. W., … Schmidtchen, A. (2018). Studies on the proteome of human hair: Identification of histones and deamidated keratins. *Scientific Reports*, 8(1599), 1–11.

Aiello, A., Tesi, A., Pratto, F., & Pierro, A. (2017). Social dominance and interpersonal power: Asymmetrical relationships within hierarchy-enhancing and hierarchy-attenuating work environments. *Journal of Applied Social Psychology*, 48(1). Retrieved from https://doi.org/10.1111/jasp.12488

American Psychiatric Association. (2013). *Diagnostic and statistical manual of mental disorders*. 5th edition. Washington, DC: American Psychiatric Press.

American Psychological Association. (2015). *Guidelines on trauma competencies for education and training*. Retrieved from: www.apa.org/ed/resources/trauma-competencies-training.pdf

Anasuri, S. (2016). Building resilience during life stages: Current status and strategies. *International Journal of Humanities and Social Science*, 6(3), 1–9.

Anda, R. (n.d.) The adverse childhood experiences study: Child abuse and public health. Prevent Child Abuse America. Retrieved from www.preventchildabuse.org/images/docs/anda_wht_ppr.pdf

Anda, R. F., Brown, D. W., Felitti, V. J., Dube, S. R., & Giles, W. H. (2008). Adverse childhood experiences and prescription drug use in a cohort study of adult HMO clients. *BMC Public Health*, 8(198), 1–9.

Anda, R., & Felitti, V. (2008). The relationship of adverse childhood experiences to adult health, well-being, social function, and healthcare. Retrieved from http://citeseerx.ist.psu.edu/viewdoc/download?doi=10.1.1.545.278&rep=rep1&type=pdf

Anda, R. F., Felitti, V.J., Bremner, J. D., Walker, J. D., Whitfield, C., … Perry, B. D. (2006). The enduring effects of abuse and related adverse experiences of childhood: A convergence of evidence from neurobiology and epidemiology. *European Archives for Psychiatry and Clinical Neuroscience*, 256(3), 174–186.

Andermahr, S. (2015). Decolonizing trauma studies: Trauma and postcolonialism—Introduction. *Humanities*, 4, 500–505.

Andersen, S. L. (2015). Exposure to early adversity: Points of cross-species translation that can lead to improved understanding of depression. *Development and Psychopathology*, 27(2), 477–491.

Anderson, E., Blitz, L., & Saastamoinen, M. (2015). Exploring a school–university model for professional development with classroom staff: Teaching trauma-informed approaches. *School Community Journal*, 25(2), 113–134.

Andolina, D., di Segni, M., & Ventura, R. (2017). MiRNA-34 and stress response. *Oncotarget*, 8(4), 5658–5659.

Andrews, A., Jobe-Shields, L., López, C., & Metzger, I. (2015). Polyvictimization, income, and ethnic differences in trauma-related mental health during adolescence. *Social Psychiatry Psychiatric Epidemiology*, 50(8), 1223–1234.

Anthony, E. (2017). Risk and resilience. Retrieved from www.oxfordbibliographies. com/view/docum ent/obo-9780199791231/obo-9780199791231–0147.xml

Arditti, J. (2012). Child trauma within the context of parental incarceration: A family process perspective. *Journal of Family Theory and Review*, 4(3), 181–219.

Aschrafi, A., Verheijen, J., Gordebeke, P., Loohuis, N., Menting, K., Jager, A. … Kozicz, T. (2016). MicroRNA-326 acts as a molecular switch in the regulation of midbrain urocortin 1 expression. *Journal of Psychiatry & Neuroscience: JPN*, 41(5), 342–353.

Avillion, A., & Hamilton, P. (2018). Burnout and stresscreating a healthy workplace. Retrieved from http://www.nursingceu.com/courses/494/index_nceu.html

Baker, F. A., Metcalf, O., Varker, T., & O'Donnell, M. (2017, December 4). A systematic review of the efficacy of creative arts therapies in the treatment of adults with PTSD. *Psychological Trauma: Theory, Research, Practice, and Policy*. Advance online publication. Retrieved from http://dx.doi.org/10.1037/tra0000353

Balistreri, K. S. (2015). Adverse childhood experiences, the medical home, and child well- being. *Maternal and Child Health Journal*, 19(11), 2492–2500.

Balistreri, K. S., & Alvira-Hammond, M. (2016). Adverse childhood experiences, family functioning and adolescent health and emotional well-being. *Public Health*, 132, 72–78.

Baran, N. M. (2017). Sensitive periods, vasotocin-family peptides, and the evolution and development of social behavior. *Frontiers in Endocrinology*, 8, 189. Retrieved from http://doi.org/10.3389/fendo.2017.00189

Barchitta, M., Maugeri, A., Quattrocchi, A., Agrifoglio, O., & Agodi, A. (2017). The role of miRNAs as biomarkers for pregnancy outcomes: A comprehensive review. *International Journal of Genomics*. Retrieved from http://doi.org/10.1155/2017/8067972

Barrera, I. (2008). An ecological systems theory approach in looking at mental health care barriers in the Latino Community. Retrieved from http://citeseerx.ist.psu.edu/viewdoc/download?doi=10.1.1.625.8819&rep=rep1&type=pdf

Bauerly, B. (2018). Integrating trauma-informed practices across state government: The Wisconsin way. *The Network for Public Health Law*. Retrieved from www.networkforphl.org/the_network_blog/2018/01/31/961/integrating_trauma- informed_practices_across_state_government_the_wisconsin_way

Becker-Blease, K. (2017). As the world becomes trauma-informed, work to do. *Journal of Trauma & Dissociation*, 18(2), 131–138.

Bellis, M., Hughes, K., Hardcastle, K., Ashton, K., Ford, K., Quigg, Z., & Davies, A. (2017). The impact of adverse childhood experiences on health service use across the life course using a retrospective cohort study. *Journal of Health Services Research & Policy*, 22(3), 168–177.

Berg, J., Osher, D., Moroney, D., Yoder, N. (2017). The intersection of school climate and social and emotional development. American Institutes for Research. Retrieved from www.air.org/sites/default/files/downloads/report/Intersection-School-Climate-and-Social-and-Emotional-Development-February-2017.pdf

Berger, R., & Quiros, L. (2014). Supervision for trauma-informed practice. *Traumatology*, 20(4), 296–301.

Beutel, M., Tibubos, A., Klein, E., Schmutzer, G., Reiner, I., & Brahler, E. (2017). Childhood adversities and distress – The role of resilience in a representative sample. *PlosONE*. Retrieved from http://journals.plos.org/plosone/article?id=10.1371/journal.pone.0173826

Bick, J., & Nelson, C. A. (2016). Early adverse experiences and the developing brain. *Neuropsychopharmacology*, 41(1), 177–196.

Bielenberg, J., Garcia, C., Henley, C., Lin, A., Martinez, B., & Weiler, A. (2015). Adverse childhood experiences, trauma informed care and resilience: Findings, policies and assessments. Retrieved from www.wellspringpacific.org/uploads/5/8/7/9/587 97525/pacific_county_aces_report.pdf

Bierman, K. L. (2004). *Peer Rejection: Developmental Processes and Intervention Strategies.* New York: Guilford.

Biglan, A., Van Ryzin, M., & Hawkins, J. (2017). Evolving a more nurturing society to prevent adverse childhood experiences. *Academic Pediatrics*, 17(7S), S150–S157.

Black, M. M., Walker, S. P., Fernald, L. C. H., Andersen, C. T., DiGirolamo, A. M., Lu, C., ... for the Lancet Early Childhood Development Series Steering Committee. (2017). Early childhood development coming of age: Science through the life course. *Lancet*, 389(10064), 77–90.

Blanch, A., Shern, D., Steverman, S. (2014). Toxic stress, behavioral health, and the next major era in public health. *Mental Health America*. Retrieved from www.mentalhealthamerica.net/issues/toxic-stress-behavioral-health-and-next-major-era-public-health

Blankenship, D. M. (2017). Five efficacious treatments for posttraumatic stress disorder: An empirical review. *Journal of Mental Health Counseling*, 39(4), 275–288.

Blaze, J., Asok, A., & Roth, T. L. (2015). The long-term impact of adverse caregiving environments on epigenetic modifications and telomeres. *Frontiers in Behavioral Neuroscience*, 9, 79, doi: doi:10.3389/fnbeh.2015.00079

Blitz, L. V., Anderson, E. M., & Saastamoinen, M. (2016). Assessing perceptions of culture and trauma in an elementary school: Informing a model for culturally responsive trauma- informed schools. *The Urban Review*, 48(4), 520–542.

Bloom, S. L. (1997). *Creating sanctuary: Toward the evolution of sane societies* (1st edition). New York: Routledge.

Bloom, S. L. (2000). Origins of international society for traumatic stress studies. In A. Shalev, R. Yehuda, & A. McFarlane (Eds.), *International handbook of human response to trauma* (27–50). New York: Plenum Publishing.

Bloom, S. L. (2013). The impact of trauma on development and well-being. Retrieved from www.sanctuaryweb.com/Portals/0/Bloom%20Pubs/2013%20Bloom%20The%20Impact%20of%20Trauma%20on%20Development%20and%20Well-being.pdf

Bloom, S. L. (2015). Trauma-informed, trauma-responsive, trauma-specific. Retrieved from http://sanctuaryweb.com/News.aspx

Bloom, S. L. (2016). Advancing a national cradle-to-grave-tocradle public health agenda. *Journal of Trauma & Dissociation*, 17(4), 383–396.

Bloom, S. L. (2017). Healthy systems—trauma informed and trauma responsive. Retrieved from http://marc.healthfederation.org/sites/default/files/Bloom_Healthy%20Systems%20are%20TI%20and%20TR_2017-06-14.pdf

Boon, H. J., Millar, J., Lake, D., Cottrell, A., & King, D. (2012). *Recovery from disaster: Resilience, adaptability and perceptions of climate change, national climate change adaptation research facility*, Final Report. National Climate Change Adaptation Research Facility, Gold Coast, Australia. Retrieved from https://researchoutput.csu.edu.au/ws/portalfiles/portal/10192546

Botha, A. (2014). *The influence of risk and resilience factors on the life satisfaction of adolescents.* PhD thesis. University of the Free State, Bloemfontein, South Africa. Retrieved from www.researchgate.net/profile/Anja_Botha/publication/281437548_The_influence_of_risk_and_resilience_factors_on_the_life_satisfaction_of_adolescents/links/55e6cf5a08ae6cf8e1331575/The-influence-of-risk-and-resilience-factors-on-the-life-satisfaction-of-adolescents.pdf

Bowen, E. A., & Murshid, N. S. (2016). Trauma-informed social policy: A conceptual framework for policy analysis and advocacy. *American Journal of Public Health*, 106(2), 223–229.

Bowlby, J. (1982). *Attachment and loss. Volume I: Attachment* (2nd edition). New York: Basic Books.

Branson, C. E., Baetz, C. L., Horwitz, S. M., & Hoagwood, K. E. (2017, February 6). Trauma-informed juvenile justice systems: A systematic review of definitions and core components. *Psychological Trauma: Theory, Research, Practice, and Policy*, 9(6), 635–646.

Braveman, P., & Gottlieb, L. (2014). The social determinants of health: It's time to consider the causes of the causes. *Public Health Reports*, 129(Suppl 2), 19–31.

Brendtro, L. K. (2015). Our resilient brain: Nature's most complex creation. *Reclaiming Children and Youth*, 24(2), 41–49.

Brendtro, L. K., & Mitchell, M. L. (2014). Powerful outcomes: Delivering what works. *Reclaiming Children and Youth*, 22(4), 5–11.

Breslau, N., Wilcox, H., Storr, C., Lucia, V., & Anthony, J. (2004). Trauma exposure and posttraumatic stress disorder: A study of youths in urban America. *Journal of Urban Health*, 81, 530–544.

Briggs-Gowan, M., Carter, A., Clark, R., Augustyn, M., McCarthy, K., & Ford, J. (2010). Exposure to potentially traumatic events in early childhood: Differential links to emergent psychopathology. *Journal of Child Psychology and Psychiatry*, 51, 1132–1140.

Brodowski, M., & Fischman, L. (2013). Protective factors for populations served by the administration on children, youth, and families. Retrieved from www.dsgonline. com/acyf/DSG%20Protective% 20Factors%20Literature%20Revie w%202013.pdf

Browne, A., Varcoe, C., Lavoie, J., Smye, V., Wong, S., Krause, M. … Fridkin, A. (2016). Enhancing health care equity with Indigenous populations: Evidence-based strategies from an ethnographic study. *BMC Health Services Research*, 16, 544–562.

Brous, K. (2014). Developmental trauma: What you can't see? Can hurt you… *ACEs Connection*. Retrieved from www.acesconnection.com/blog/developmental- trauma-what-you-can-t-see-can-hurt-you

Bruder, M. (2013). Factors influencing family medicine residents' screening for intimate partner violence. Indiana State University, Terre Haute, IN. Retrieved from http://scholars.indstate.edu/ha ndle/10484/5470

Brumley, L. D., Jaffee, S. R., & Brumley, B. P. (2017). Pathways from childhood adversity to problem behaviors in young adulthood: The mediating role of adolescents' future expectations. *Journal of Youth and Adolescence*, 46(1), 1–14.

Bruner, C. (2017). ACE, place, race, and poverty: Building hope for children. *Academic Pediatrics*, 17 (7S), S123–S129. Retrieved from www.academicpedsjnl.net/article/S1876-2859(17)30352-2/fulltext

Brunzell, T., Stokes, H., & Waters, L. (2016). Trauma-informed positive education: Using positive psychology to strengthen vulnerable students. *Contemporary School Psychology*, 20, 63–83.

Buck, P., Bean, N., & de Marco, K. (2017). Equine-assisted psychotherapy: An emerging trauma-informed intervention. *Advances in Social Work*, 18(1), 387–402.

Buckminster Fuller Institute. (n. d.). Greenwave. Retrieved from https://www.bfi.org/Ideaindex/projects/ 2015/greenwave

Bywaters, P., Bunting, L., Davidson, G., Hanratty, J.Mason, W., McCartan, C., & Steils, N. (2016). *The relationship between poverty, child abuse and neglect: An evidence review*. York, UK: Joseph Rowntree Foundation. Retrieved from www.researchgate.net/publication/295812966_The_relationship_ between_poverty_child_abuse_and_neglect_an_evidence_review

Callaghan, B. L., & Tottenham, N. (2016). The stress acceleration hypothesis: Effects of early-life adversity on emotion circuits and behavior. *Current Opinion in Behavioral Sciences*, 7, 76–81.

Candib, L., Savageau, J., Weinreb, L., & Reed, G. (2012). Inquiring into our past: When the doctor is a survivor of abuse. *Family Medicine and Community Health Publications and Presentations*, 44(6), 416–424. Retrieved from https://escholarship.umassmed.edu/fmch_articles/226

Capatosto, K. (2015). *From punitive to restorative: Advantages of using trauma-informed practices in schools*. Columbus, OH: Kirwan Institute. Retrieved from http://kirwaninstitute.osu.edu/wp-content/uploa ds/2016/04/From-Punitive-to-Restorative1.pdf

Carello, J., & Butler, L. (2015). Practicing what we teach: Trauma informed educational practice. *Journal of Teaching in Social Work*, 35(3), 262–278.

Caven, K. (2018, March 14). Oprah learns about ACEs and trauma-informed care. *ACEs too High*. Retrieved from https://acestoohigh.com/2018/03/14/this-changed-my-life-oprah-learns-about-a ces-and-trauma-informed-care/

Centers for Disease Control and Prevention (CDC). (2010). Adverse childhood experiences reported by adults—Five states, 2009. Morbidity and Mortality Weekly Report, 59(49), 1609–1613.

Centers for Disease Control and Prevention (CDC). (2016). About the CDC-Kaiser ACE study: Study questionnaires. Retrieved from www.cdc.gov/violenceprevention/acestudy/about.html

Chafouleas, S., Johnson, A., Overstreet, S., & Santos, N. (2016). Toward a blueprint for trauma-informed service delivery in schools. *School Mental Health: A Multidisciplinary Research and Practice Journal*, 8(1), 144–162.

Chamberlain, L. J., Hanson, E. R., Klass, P., Schickedanz, A., Nakhasi, A., Barnes, M. M., Berger, S., Boyd, R. W., Dreyer, B. P., Meyer, D., Navsaria, D., Rao, S., & Klein, M. (2016). Childhood poverty and its effect on health and well-being: Enhancing training for learners across the medical education continuum. *Academic Pediatrics*, 16(3S), S155–S162.

Chapman, D. P., Whitfield, C. L., Felitti, V. J., Dube, S. R., Edwards, V. J., & Anda, R. F. (2004). Adverse childhood experiences and the risk of depressive disorders in adulthood. *Journal of Affective Disorders*, 82(2), 217–225

Chen, R., Gillespie, A., Zhao, Y., Xi, Y., Ren, Y., & McLean, L. (2018). The efficacy of eye movement desensitization and reprocessing in children and adults who have experienced complex childhood trauma: A systematic review of randomized controlled trials. *Frontiers in Psychology*, 9, (534).

Chilton, M. (2018). 'What happened' vs. 'what's wrong': Recognizing how trauma impacts us all. *The Inquirer*. Retrieved from www.philly.com/philly/opinion/commentary/trauma-oprah-60-minutes-what-happened-to-you-opinion-20180315.html

Cicchetti, D., & Andersen, S. L. (2015). Exposure to early adversity: Points of cross-species translation that can lead to improved understanding of depression. *Development and Psychopathology*, 27(2), 477–491.

Cicchetti, D., Georgieff, M. K., Brunette, K. E., & Tran, P. V. (2015). Early life nutrition and neural plasticity. *Development and Psychopathology*, 27(2), 411–423.

Clervil, R., & DeCandia, C. (2013). *Integrating and sustaining trauma-informed care across diverse service systems*. The National Center on Family Homelessness at the American Institutes for Research. Retrieved from www.fredla.org/wp-content/uploads/2016/01/Tap-Trauma-informed-Systems-of-Care-Brief_092713_Ack.pdf

Cless, J. D., & Nelson-Goff, B. S. (2017). Teaching trauma: A model for introducing traumatic materials in the classroom. *Advances in Social Work*, 18(1), 25–38.

Cohen, L., Davis, R., & Realini, A. (2016). Communities are not all created equal: Strategies to prevent violence affecting youth in the United States. *Journal of Public Health Policy*, 37 (Suppl 1), 81–94.

Conley, D., & Malaspina, D. (2016). Socio-genomics and structural competency. *Bioethical Inquiry*, 13, 193–202.

Courtois, C., & Gold, S. (2009). The need for inclusion of psychological trauma in the professional curriculum: A call to action. *Psychological Trauma: Theory, Research, Practice, and Policy*, 1(1), 3–23.

Cronholm, P., Forke, C., Wade, R., Bair-Merritt, M., Davis, M., Harkins-Schwartz, M., Pachter, L., & Fein, J. (2015). Adverse childhood experiences expanding the concept of adversity. *American Journal of Preventive Medicine*, 49(3), 354–361.

Czyzewski, K. (2011). Colonialism as a broader social determinant of health. *The International Indigenous Policy Journal*, 2(5), 1–17.

Danese, A., & Baldwin, J. (2017). Hidden wounds? Inflammatory links between childhood trauma and psychopathology. *Annual Review of Psychology*, 68, 517–544.

Dauber, S., Lotsos, K., & Pulido, M. L. (2015). Treatment of complex trauma on the front lines: A preliminary look at child outcomes in an agency sample. *Child & Adolescent Social Work Journal*, 32(6), 529–543.

Davis, M., Costigan, T., & Schubert, K. (2017). Promoting lifelong health and well-being: Staying the course to promote health and prevent the effects of adverse childhood and community experiences. *Academic Pediatrics*, 17, S4–S6.

De Bellis, M., & Zisk, A. (2014). The biological effects of childhood trauma. *Child and Adolescent Psychiatric Clinics of North America*, 23(2), 185–222.

DeCandia, C., & Guarino, K. (2015). Trauma informed care: An ecological response. *Journal of Child and Youth Care Work*, 25, 7–32. Retrieved from www.air.org/sites/default/files/downloads/report/Trauma-Informed-Care-An-Ecological-Response-Guarino-2015.pdf

DeCandia, C., Guarino, K., & Clervil, R. (2014). *Trauma-informed care and trauma-specific services: A comprehensive approach to trauma intervention.* American Institutes for Research. Retrieved from www.air.org/sites/default/files/downloads/report/Trauma-Informed%20Care%20White%20Paper_October%202014.pdf

Defending Childhood Initiative. (2013). Defending childhood: Protect, heal, thrive. Retrieved from www.juvenilecouncil.gov/materials/2015_11/Handout_Defending_Childhood_2_pager_updated_may_2013.pdf

DeLisi, M., & Vaughn, M. (2015). The vindication of Lamarck? Epigenetics at the intersection of law and mental health. *Behavorial Sciences and the Law*, 33(5), 607–628.

De Sanctis, V., Nomura, Y., Newcorn, J., & Halperin, J. (2012). Childhood maltreatment and conduct disorder: Independent predictors of criminal outcomes in ADHD youth. *Child Abuse & Neglect*, 36 (11–12), 782–789.

de Zulueta, P. C. (2015). Developing compassionate leadership in health care: an integrative review. *Journal of Healthcare Leadership*, 8, 1–10. doi:10.2147/JHL.S93724

de Zulueta, P. (2016). Developing compassionate leadership in health care: An integrative review. *Journal of Healthcare Leadership*, 8, 1–10.

Dias, B. G., Maddox, S., Klengel, T., & Ressler, K. J. (2015). Epigenetic mechanisms underlying learning and the inheritance of learned behaviors. *Trends in Neuroscience*, 38(2), 96–107.

Dowd, M. D. (2017). Early adversity, toxic stress, and resilience: Pediatrics for today. *Pediatric Annals*, 46 (7), e246–e249.

Dressler, W. (2001). Medical anthropology: Toward a third moment in social science? *Medical Anthropology Quarterly*, 15(4), 455–465.

Drexel University (2018). Trauma-informed care course. Retrieved from http://catalog.drexel.edu/search/?P=BACS%20380

Drury, S. S., Sánchez, M. M., & Gonzalez, A. (2016). When mothering goes awry: Challenges and opportunities for utilizing evidence across rodent, nonhuman primate and human studies to better define the biological consequences of negative early caregiving. *Hormones and Behavior*, 77, 182–192.

Dube, S. R., Anda, R. F., Felitti, V. J., Edwards, V. J., & Croft, J. B. (2002). Adverse childhood experiences and personal alcohol abuse as an adult. *Addictive Behaviors*, 27(5), 713–725.

Dube, S. R., Felitti, V. J., Dong, M., Chapman, D. P., Giles, W. H., & Anda, R. F. (2003). Childhood abuse, neglect, and household dysfunction and the risk of illicit drug use: The adverse childhood experiences study. *Pediatrics*, 111(3), 564–572.

Dube, S. R., Miller, J. W., Brown, D. W., Giles, W. H., Felitti, V. J., Dong, M., & Anda, R. F. (2006). Adverse childhood experiences and the association with ever using alcohol and initiating alcohol use during adolescence. *Journal of Adolescent Health*, 38(4), 444.e1– 444.e10.

Dudley, R. (2015). Childhood Trauma and Its Effects: Implications for Police. *New Perspectives in Policing*, 1–22, Retrieved from www.ncjrs.gov/pdffiles1/nij/248686.pdf

Edalati, H., Nicholls, T., Crocker, A., Somers, J., & Patterson, M. (2017). Adverse childhood experiences and the risk of criminal justice involvement and victimization among homeless adults with mental illness. *Psychiatric Services*, 68(12),1288–1295.

Edmonds, G. W., Hampson, S. E., Côté, H. C. F., Hill, P. L., & Klest, B. (2016). Childhood personality, betrayal trauma, and leukocyte telomere length in adulthood: A lifespan perspective on conscientiousness and betrayal traumas as predictors of a biomarker of cellular aging. *European Journal of Personality*, 30(5), 426–437.

Ellis, W., & Dietz, W. (2017). A new framework for addressing adverse childhood and community experiences: The building community resilience model. *Academic Pediatrics*, 17(7), S86–S93.

ENCODE Project Consortium. (2012). An integrated encyclopedia of DNA elements in the human genome. *Nature*, 489(7414), 57–74.

Essen, C., Freshwater, D., & Cahill, J. (2015). Towards an understanding of the dynamic sociomaterial embodiment of interprofessional collaboration. *Nursing Inquiry*, 22, 210–220.

Fairbrother, G., Dougherty, D., Pradhananga, R., & Simpson, L. (2017). Road to the future: Priorities for child health services research. *Academic Pediatrics*, 17(8), 814–824.

Fallot, R., & Harris, M. (2001). Culture shock. *National Council Magazine*. Retrieved from www.thena tionalcouncil.org/wp-content/uploads/2012/11/NC-Mag-Trauma-Web-Email.pdf

Fallot, R. D., & Harris, M. (2002). The Trauma Recovery and Empowerment Model (TREM): Conceptual and practical issues in a group intervention for women. *Community Mental Health Journal*, 38(6), 475–485.

Fallot, R. D., & Harris, M. (2009). Creating cultures of trauma-informed care (CCTIC): A self-assessment and planning protocol. Retrieved from www.theannainstitute.org/CCTICSELFASSPP.pdf

Family and Children Services (2018). Family & children services join community-wide effort to break generational cycle of adverse childhood experiences. Retrieved from www.fcsource.org/Agency_News_article17-12c.html

Felitti, V. (2002). The relation between adverse childhood experiences and adult health: Turning gold into lead. *The Permanente Journal*, 6(1), 44–47. Retrieved from www.ncbi.nlm.nih.gov/pmc/articles/PMC6220625/

Felitti, V., Anda, R., Nordenberg, D., Williamson, D., Spitz, A., Edwards, V., Koss, M., & Marks, J. (1998). Relationship of childhood abuse and household dysfunction to many of the leading causes of death in adults. *American Journal of Preventive Medicine*, 14(4), 245–258.

Felter, J., & Ayers, L. (2016). Incorporating trauma informed practice and ACEs into professional curricula: A toolkit. Retrieved from http://mindpeacecincinnati.com/wp-content/uploads/Incorpora ting-Trauma-Informed-Practice-and-ACEs-into-Professional-Curricula-a-Toolkit.pdf

Feuer-Edwards, A., O'Brien, C., & O'Connor, S. (2016). Trauma-informed philanthropy. Retrieved from https://c.ymcdn.com/sites/www.philanthropynetwork.org/resource/resmgr/pn_miscdocs/Tra umaGUIDE_FinalWeb.pdf

Fink, D. S., & Galea, S. (2015). Life course epidemiology of trauma and related psychopathology in civilian populations. *Current Psychiatry Reports*, 17(5), 1–16.

Finkelhor, D., Shattuck, A., Turner, H., & Hamby, S. (2013). Improving the adverse childhood experiences study scale. *JAMA Pediatrics*, 167(1), 70–75.

Fiori, L., & Turecki, G. (2016). Investigating epigenetic consequences of early-life adversity: Some methodological considerations, *European Journal of Psychotraumatology*, 7(1), 1–9.

Flaherty, E. G., Thompson, R., Dubowitz, H., Harvey, E. M., English, D. J., Everson, M. D., … Runyan, D. K. (2013). Adverse childhood experiences and child health in early adolescence. *JAMA Pediatrics*, 167(7), 622–629.

Florin, M.-V., & Linkov, I. (Eds.). (2016). *IRGC resource guide on resilience*. Lausanne, Switzerland: EPFL International Risk Governance Center (IRGC). Retrieved from https://infoscience.epfl.ch/record/228206/files/IRGC.%20(2016).%20Resource%20guide%20on%20resilience.%20Book.pdf

Ford, E. S., Zhao, G., Tsai, J., & Li, C. (2011). Low-risk lifestyle behaviors and all-cause mortality: Findings from the national health and nutrition examination survey III mortality study. *American Journal of Public Health*, 101(10), 1922–1929.

Forge, N., Hartinger-Saunders, R., Wright, E., & Ruel, E. (2018). Out of the system and onto the streets: LGBTQ-identified youth experiencing homelessness with past child welfare system involvement. *Child Welfare*, 96(2), 47–74.

Freeman, J. (2017). The child is father of the man: Family physicians' screening for adverse childhood experiences. *Family Medicine*, 49(1), 5–6.

Fulford, W. (2017). Hidden suffering and the effects of adverse childhood experiences. *Religions*, 8(3), 1–8. Retrieved from www.mdpi.com/2077-1444/8/3/31/htm

Garbarino, J. (2017). ACEs in the criminal justice system. *Academic Pediatric*, 17(7), S32–S33.

Garner, A. S. (2016). Thinking developmentally: The next evolution in models of health. *Journal of Developmental & Behavioral Pediatrics*, 37(7), 579–584.

Gaskill, R., & Perry, B. (2014). The neurobiological power of play using the neurosequential model of therapeutics to guide play in the healing process. In C. A. Malchiodi & D. A. Crenshaw (Eds.), *Creative arts and play therapy for attachment problems* (178–194). New York: Guilford Press. Retrieved from https://childtrauma.org/wp-content/uploads/2014/12/Malchiodi_Perry_Gaskill.pdf

Geronimus, A., Bound, J., & Colen, C. (2011). Excess lack mortality in the United States and in selected black and white high-poverty areas, 1980–2000. *American Journal of Public Health*, 101(4), 720–729.

Gerson, R., & Corwin, D. (2015). The cost of adverse childhood experiences. In D. Corwin (Ed.), *Adverse childhood experiences: Informing best practices* (58–60). Jacksonville, FL: Academy on Violence and Abuse (AVA). Retrieved from www.avahealth.org/file_download/aee3fd13-8ab5-460a-8a e7-4cc054a2c331

Gilbert, L., Breiding, M., Merrick, M., Thompson, W., Ford, D., Dhingra, S., & Parks, S. (2015). Childhood adversity and adult chronic disease: An update from ten states and the District of Columbia, 2010. *American Journal of Preventive Medicine*, 48(3), 345–349.

Gilgun, J., & Hirschey, S. (2017). A four-factor outcome model for family case management services with children and families who have experienced complex trauma. *Journal of Family Theory & Review*, 9(4), 537–556.

Gillihan, S. (2018). Why can't I get over my painful childhood? *Psychology Today*. Retrieved from www.psychologytoday.com/us/blog/think-act-be/201803/why-cant-i-get-over-my-pa inful-childhood

Gilliver, C. (2016). Arts & trauma informed care within homelessness services: the development of arts-based cooperatives as a route into employment. Retrieved from https://www.wcmt.org.uk/sites/ default/files/report-documents/Gilliver%20C%20Report%202016%20Revised.pdf

Giordano, A. L., Prosek, E. A., Stamman, J., Callahan, M. M., Loseu, S., Bevly, C. M., … Chadwell, K. (2016). Addressing trauma in substance abuse treatment. *Journal of Alcohol and Drug Education*, 60 (2), 55–71.

Girouard, S., & Bailey, N. (2017). ACEs implications for nurses, nursing education, and nursing practice. *Academic Pediatrics*, 17(7), S16–S17.

Gómez, J. M., Lewis, J. K., Noll, L. K., Smidt, A. M., & Birrell, P. J. (2016). Shifting the focus: Nonpathologizing approaches to healing from betrayal trauma through an emphasis on relational care. *Journal of Trauma & Dissociation*, 17(2), 165–185.

Goodreads. (2018). Bessel A. van der Kolk. Retrieved from www.goodreads.com/quotes/7672346-a s-long-as-you-keep-secrets-and-suppress-information-you

Goodreads. (2019). Mother Teresa. Retrieved from https://www.goodreads.com/quotes/ 441072-the-way-you-help-heal-the-world-is-you-start

Green, J. G., McLaughlin, K. A., Berglund, P. A., Gruber, M. l. J., Sampson, N. A., Zaslavsky, A. M., & Kessler, R. C. (2010). Childhood adversities and adult psychiatric disorders in the national comorbidity survey replication I: Associations with first onset of DSM-IV disorders. *Archives of General Psychiatry*, 67(2), 113–123.

Greer, T. (2017). Racial-trauma informed ministry: A process for dominant culture ministries to effectively engage with communities impacted by racial trauma. *Seattle Pacific Seminary Projects*, 4. Retrieved from http://digitalcommons.spu.edu/spseminary_projects/4

Greyber, L. R., Dulmus, C. N., Cristalli, M., & Jorgensen, J. (2015). A single group pre-posttest examination of a health and wellness intervention on body mass index for adolescent females with severe emotional disorders and histories of trauma. *Child & Adolescent Social Work Journal*, 32(2), 187–198.

Guardian. (2014). Maya Angelou quotes: 15 of the best. Retrieved from https://www.theguardian. com/books/2014/may/28/maya-angelou-in-fifteen-quotes

Guarino, K., Clervil, R., & Beach, C. (2014). *Trauma-informed care for veterans experiencing homelessness*. Washington, DC: American Institutes for Research. Retrieved from www.air.org/sites/default/files/ Trauma-informed%20care%20for%20homeless%20veterans%20Building%20Workforce%20Capacity %20Nov%202014.pdf

Gulliver, T., & Campney, A. (2015). Healing the pain and hurt: Dealing with the trauma of homelessness. Homelessness is only one piece of the puzzle. In The Inclusion Working Group Canadian Observatory on Homelessness (Eds.), *Homelessness is only one piece of my puzzle: Implications for policy and practice* (136–151). Toronto, ON: The Homeless Hub Press. Retrieved from https://homeles

shub.ca/sites/default/files/Homelessness%20Is%20Only%20One%20Piece%20Of%20My%20Puzzle% 20-%20Web%20V2_0.pdf#page=143

Halfon, N. (2016). Poverty, complexity, and a new way forward. *Academic Pediatrics*, 6(3), S16–S18.

Halfon, N., Larson, K., Lu, M., Tullis, E., & Russ, S. (2014). Lifecourse health development: Past, present and future. *Maternal and Child Health*, 18(2), 344–365.

Halfon, N., Larson, K., Son, J., Lu, M., & Bethell, C. (2017). Income inequality and the differential effect of adverse childhood experiences in US children. *Academic Pediatrics*, 17(7), S70–S78.

Hall, C., & Spencer, R. (2017). Illuminating the phenomenological challenges of cross-cultural supervision. *Smith Studies in Social Work*, 87(2–3), 238–253.

Han, S. (2017). ACEs in the news: How can advocates communicate more effectively about childhood trauma? *Bmsg blog.* Retrieved from http://mediastudiesgroup.com/blog/adverse-childhood-experien ces-trauma-news-communication

Handran, J. (2013). Trauma-informed organizational culture: The prevention, reduction and treatment of compassion fatigue. PhD thesis. Colorado State University. Retrieved from https://dspace.library. colostate.edu/bitstream/handle/10217/78825/Handran_colostate_0053A_11673.pdf?sequence=1

Hartley, C. A., & Lee, F. S. (2015). Sensitive periods in affective development: Nonlinear maturation of fear learning. *Neuropsychopharmacology*, 40(1), 50–60.

Haynes, A., Cuthbert, C., Gardner, R., Telford, P., & Hodson, D. (2015). *Thriving communities: A framework for preventing and intervening early in child neglect*. NSPCC. Retrieved from www.staffsscb.org. uk/Aboutus/Priorites-2012-2013/Neglect-and-the-Toxic-Trio/thriving-communities-framewor k-neglect-report.pdf

Health Resources and Services Administration. (2017). School-based health centers. Retrieved from www.hrsa.gov/our-stories/school-health-centers/index.html

Heffernan, T., Todorow, M., & Luu, H. (2015, July 7). Why housing first won't end homelessness. *Rabble.* Retrieved from http://rabble.ca/blogs/bloggers/views-expressed/2015/07/why-hou sing-first-wont-end-homelessness

Hensch, T. (2016). The power of the infant brain. *Sci Am.* Retrieved from https://henschlab.files. wordpress.com/2016/03/hensch-final-sciam.pdf

Hesse, E., & Main, M. (2006). Frightened, threatening, and dissociative parental behavior in low-risk samples: Description, discussion, and interpretations. *Development and Psychopathology*, 18(2), 309–343.

Hodges, M., Godbout, N., Briere, J., Lanktree, C., Gilbert, A., & Kletzka, N. (2013) Cumulative trauma and symptom complexity in children: A path analysis. *Child Abuse and Neglect*, 37(11), 891–898.

Hollins, S., & Cairns, M. (2016). MicroRNA: Small RNA mediators of the brains genomic response to environmental stress. *Progress in Neurobiology*, 143, 61–81.

Hornor, G. (2017). Resilience. *Journal of Pediatric Healthcare*, 31(3), 384–390. Retrieved from www.jp edhc.org/article/S0891-5245(16)30254-1/fulltext

Hughes, M, & Tucker, W. (2018). Poverty as an adverse childhood experience. *North Carolina Medical Journal*, 79(2), 124–126.

Hunt, T. (2018). Professionals' perceptions of vicarious trauma from working with victims of sexual trauma. Walden University, Minneapolis, MI. Retrieved from https://scholarworks.waldenu.edu/ cgi/viewcontent.cgi?article=7158&context=dissertations

Infurna, F., Rivers, C., Reich, J., & Zautra, A. (2015). Childhood trauma and personal mastery: Their influence on emotional reactivity to everyday events in a community sample of middle-aged adults. *PLOSOne.* Retrieved from https://journals.plos.org/plosone/article?id=10.1371/journal.pone.0121840

Iniguez, K., & Stankowski, R. (2016). Adverse childhood experiences and health in adulthood in a rural population-based sample. *Clinical Medicine & Research*, 14(3–4), 126–137.

International Society for Traumatic Stress Studies. (2000). ISTSS best practice parameters. Retrieved from www.istss.org/ISTSS_Main/media/Documents/ISTSS_Best_Practice_Parameters1.pdf

International Society for Traumatic Stress Studies. (2018). On-line learning library. Retrieved from www.istss.org/education-research/online-learning.aspx

Jacksonville University. (2018) How nurses can avoid vicarious trauma. Retrieved from www.jackson villeu.com/blog/nursing/how-nurses-can-avoid-vicarious-trauma/

Jones, J. & Olson, K. (2018). Change in mind: Applying neurosciences to revitalize communities. Retrieved from http://goccp.maryland.gov/wp-content/uploads/2018-mcvrc-change-in-mind.pdf

Kalmakis, K., Chandler, G., Roberts, S., & Leung, K. (2016). Nurse practitioner screening for childhood adversity among adult primary care clients: A mixed-method study. *Journal of the American Association of Nurse Practitioners*, 29(1), 35–45.

Katz, A., Zerger, S., & Hwang, S. (2017) Housing first the conversation: Discourse, policy and the limits of the possible. *Critical Public Health*, 27(1), 139–147.

Kaufman, M. (2017). Social justice and the American law school today: Since we are made for love. *Seattle University Law Review*, 40. Retrieved from https://digitalcommons.law.seattleu.edu/cgi/view content.cgi?article=2433&context=sulr

Kellam, S. G., Mackenzie, A. C., Brown, C. H., Poduska, J. M., Wang, W., Wilcox, H. C. (2011). The good behavior game and the future of prevention and treatment. *Addiction Science & Clinical Practice*, 6(1), 73–84.

Kessler, R., McLaughlin, K., Green, J., Gruber, M., Sampson, N., & Zaslavsky, A. (2010). Childhood adversities and adult psychopathology in the WHO world mental health surveys. *The British Journal of Psychiatry*, 197(5), 378–385.

Kezelman, A. M., & Stavropoulos, P. (2018). *Talking about trauma: Guide to conversations and screening for health and other service providers*. Blue Knot Foundation. Retrieved from www.blueknot.org.au/Porta ls/2/Newsletter/Talking%20About%20Trauma%20Services_WEB.pdf?ver= 2018–2004–06–160830–113

Kim, E., Park, J., & Kim, B. (2016). Type of childhood maltreatment and the risk of criminal recidivism in adult probationers: A cross-sectional study. *BMC Psychiatry*, 16, 1–9. Retrieved from https://bmcp sychiatry.biomedcentral.com/track/pdf/10.1186/s12888-016-1001-8

Kim, S. (2017). Resilience in physically maltreated adolescents: Interpersonally related protective factors and gender differences. The George Washington University. Retrieved from https://pqdtopen.pro quest.com/doc/1881314883.html?FMT=AI

Kinniburgh, K. J., Blaustein, M., Spinazzola, J., & van der Kolk, B. A. (2005). Attachment, self-regulation, and competency. *Psychiatric Annals*, 35(5), 424–430.

Klengel, T., Pape, J., Binder, E., & Mehta, D. (2014). The role of DNA methylation in stress- related psychiatric disorders. *Neuropharmacology*, 80, 115–132.

Ko, S. J., Ford, J. D., Kassam-Adams, N., Berkowitz, S. J., Wilson, C., Wong, M., & Layne, C. M. (2008). Creating TI systems: Child welfare, education, first responders, health care, juvenile justice. *Professional Psychology: Research and Practice*, 39, 325–340.

Kolb, B., Mychasiuk, R., & Gibb, R. (2014). Brain development, experience, and behavior. *Pediatric Blood & Cancer*, 61(10), 1720–1723. Retrieved from www.researchgate.net/publication/259491812_ Brain_Development_Experience_and_Behavior

Kovacic, T. (2015). Generational understanding of social support, youth civic engagement and coping as aspects of resilience in socialist and post-socialist Slovenia (1980–2011). PhD thesis. National University of Ireland, Galway. Retrieved from https://aran.library.nuigalway.ie/bitstream/handle/ 10379//5513/Tanja%20Kovacic-PhD%20Thesis.pdf?sequence=1&isAllowed=y

Kuras, Y., Assaf, N., Thoma, M., Gianferante, D., Hanln, L., Chen, X., Fiksdal, A., & Rohleder, N. (2017). Blunted diurnal cortisol activity in healthy adults with childhood adversity. *Frontiers in Human Neuroscience*, 11(574), 1–8.

Lappé, M. (2016). Epigenetics, media coverage, and parent responsibilities in the post- genomic era. *Current Genetic Medicine Reports*, 4(3), 92–97.

Laugharne, J., Kullack, C., Lee, C. W., McGuire, T., Brockman, S., Drummond, P. D., & Starkstein, S. (2016). Amygdala volumetric change following Psychotherapy for posttraumatic stress disorder. *Journal of Neuropsychiatry and Clinical Neurosciences*, 28(4), 312–318.

Lawson, K., Davis, K., McHale, S., Almeida, D., Kelly, E., & King, R. (2016). Effects of workplace intervention on affective well-being in employees' children. *Developmental Psychology*, 52(5), 772–777.

Leaver, R. (2016). The future depends on what you do today—Mahatma Gandhi. *International Journal of Urological Nursing*, 10(3), 115–117.

Lee, E., Larkin, H., & Esaki, N. (2017). Exposure to community violence as a new adverse childhood experience category: Promising results and future considerations. *Families in Society: The Journal of Contemporary Social Services*, 98(1), 69–78.

Lee, C. M., Mangurian, C., Tieu, L., Ponath, C., Guzman, D., & Kushel, M. (2017). Childhood adversities associated with poor adult mental health outcomes in older homeless adults: Results from the HOPE HOME study. *The American Journal of Geriatric Psychiatry: Official Journal of the American Association for Geriatric Psychiatry*, 25(2), 107–117.

Leeman, J. (2018). Living our parents' trauma: Effects of child abuse and neglect on the next generation. Australian Catholic University. Retrieved from http://researchbank.acu.edu.au/cgi/view content.cgi?article=1664&context=theses

Leitch, L. (2017). Action steps using ACEs and trauma-informed care: A resilience model. *Health & Justice*, 5, 5–15.

Lester, B. M., Conradt, E., & Marsit, C. (2016). Introduction to the special section on epigenetics. *Child Development*, 87(1), 29–37. doi:10.1111/cdev.12489

Lewis, A. (2009). Assessing childhood trauma: A holistic perspective. *Child Abuse Research: A South African Journal*, 10(1), 14–26.

Listenbee, R., Torre, J., Boyle, G., Cooper, S., Deanne, S., & Taguba, A. (2012). *Report of the Attorney General's National Task Force on Children Exposed to Violence*. Retrieved from https://sph.umd.edu/sites/default/files/files/cev-rpt-full.pdf

Lo, C.-L., & Zhou, F. C. (2014). Environmental alterations of epigenetics prior to the birth. *International Review of Neurobiology*, 115, 1–49.

Loi, M., Del Savio, L., & Stupka, E. (2013). Social epigenetics and equality of opportunity. *Public Health Ethics*, 6(2), 142–153.

López, C. M., Andrews, A. R., III, Chisolm, A. M., de Arellano, M. A., Saunders, B., & Kilpatrick, D. (2017). Racial/ethnic differences in trauma exposure and mental health disorders in adolescents. *Cultural Diversity and Ethnic Minority Psychology*, 23(3), 382–387.

Loveland, K. (2017). Trauma-informed approaches. Retrieved from https://mthcf.org/wp-content/uploads/2018/01/Trauma-Informed-Approaches-Brief.pdf

Luest, H. (2017). Trauma informed pioneers: First ladies working to heal communities. Retrieved from www.huffpost.com/entry/trauma-informed-pioneers-first-ladies-working-to-heal_b_58cc1c23e4b0537abd95703f

Lundberg, M. & Wuermli, A. (2012). Children and youth in crisis. The World Bank. Retrieved from https://scholar.harvard.edu/files/lamont/files/a_conceptual_framework.pdf

Lyles, A., Davis, R., Cohen, L., & Lester, L. (2017). *A good solution solves multiple problems: Exploring prevention strategies that address multiple forms of violence*. Prevention Institute. Retrieved from www.preventioninstitute.org/sites/default/files/publications/A%20Good%20Solution1%20PI%20Format%20-%20FINAL.pdf

Lyons-Ruth, K. & Jacobvitz, D. (2008) Attachment disorganization: Genetic factors, parenting contexts, and developmental transformations from infancy to adulthood. In: Cassidy, J. and Shaver, P.R., Eds., *Handbook of attachment. Theory, research, and clinical applications*. New York: Guilford Press, 666–697.

Macdonald, A., Danielson, C., Resnick, H., Saunders, B., & Kilpatrick, D. (2010). PTSD and comorbid disorders in a representative sample of adolescents: The risk associated with multiple exposures to potentially traumatic events. *Child Abuse and Neglect*, 34(10), 773–783.

Make It So. (2016). *Healthy families: From ACEs to trauma-informed care to resilience and wellbeing: Examples of policies and activities across IIMHL & IIDL countries*. Retrieved from www.iimhl.com/files/docs/Make_It_So/20161206.pdf

Mann, M. J., Kristjansson, A. L., Sigfusdottir, I. D., & Smith, M. L. (2014). The impact of negative life events on young adolescents: Comparing the relative vulnerability of middle level, high school, and college-age students. *Research in Middle Level Education Online*, 38(2), 1–13.

Mansour, J., & Curran, M. (2016). Child poverty: The united kingdom experience. *Academic Pediatrics*, 16(3), S76–S82.

Martin, C. G., Van Ryzin, M. J., & Dishion, T. J. (2016). Profiles of childhood trauma: Betrayal, frequency, and psychological distress in late adolescence. *Psychological Trauma: Theory, Research, Practice and Policy*, 8(2), 206–213.

Matta, G., Woodward-Kron, R. E., Petty, S., & Salzber, M. (2016). Eliciting and responding to patient histories of abuse and trauma: Challenges for medical education. *Medical Journal of Australia*, 205(6), 248–249.

Maunder, R. G., Peladeau, N., Savage, D., & Lancee, W. (2010). The prevalence of childhood adversity among health care workers and its relationship to adult life events, distress and impairment. *Child Abuse and Neglect*, 34, 114–123.

McCarthy, M., Taylor, P., Norman, R., Pezzullo, L., Tucci, J., & Goddard, C. (2016). The lifetime economic and social costs of child maltreatment in Australia. *Children and Youth Services Review*, 71, 217–226.

Mcchesney, G. C., Adamson, G., & Shevlin, M. (2015). A latent class analysis of trauma based on a nationally representative sample of US adolescents. *Social Psychiatry and Psychiatric Epidemiology*, 50(8), 1207–1217.

McEwen, B. S. (2017). Neurobiological and systemic effects of chronic stress. *Chronic Stress (Thousand Oaks)*, 1, 1–17.

McEwen, C., & McEwen, B. (2017). Social structure, adversity, toxic stress, and intergenerational poverty: An early childhood model. *Annual Review of Sociology*, 43(1), 445–472.

McLaughlin, K. (2016). Future directions in childhood adversity and youth psychopathology. *Journal of Clinical Child & Adolescent Psychology*, 45(3), 361–382.

McLean, C. P., Yeh, R., Rosenfield, D., & Foa, E. B. (2015). Changes in negative cognitions mediate PTSD symptom reductions during client-centered therapy and prolonged exposure for adolescents. *Behaviour Research and Therapy*, 68, 64–69.

McWhinnie, L. (2017) An interprofessional approach to trauma-informed care in the mood and anxiety program at health sciences north. Laurentian University Sudbury, Ontario. Retrieved from https://zone.biblio.laurentian.ca/bitstream/10219/2740/1/Advanced%20Practicum%20Paper-%20Lauren%20McWhinnie.pdf

Menschner, C., & Maul, A. (2016). *Key ingredients for successful trauma-informed care implementation*. Center for Health Care Strategies and the Robert Wood Johnson Foundation. Retrieved from www.chcs.org/media/ATC_whitepaper_040616.pdf

Merck, A. (2018). 5 big policy strategies to tackle childhood trauma—and a toolkit to make it happen. *Salud America!* Retrieved from https://salud-america.org/communications-toolkit-and-5-policy-recommendations-to-address-childhood-trauma/

Metzl, J. M., & Hansen, H. (2014). Structural competency: Theorizing a new medical engagement with stigma and inequality. *Social Science & Medicine*, 103, 126–133.

Metzler, M., Merrick, M., Klevens, J., Ports, K., & Ford, D. (2017). Adverse childhood experiences and life opportunities: Shifting the narrative. *Children and Youth Services Review*, 17, 141–149.

Miller, A. W., Conrad, D. V., Brady, M. J., Moffitt, M. P., & Bay, R. C. (2004). Medical student training in domestic violence: A comparison of students entering residency training in 1995 and 2001. *Teaching and Learning in Medicine*, 16, 3–6.

Mitchell, C., Schneper, L., & Notterman, D. (2016). DNA methylation, early life environment, and health outcomes. *Pediatric Research*, 79(1–2), 212–219.

Moffic, H. S. (2016). Ethics column: A new psychiatric administrative ethical challenge: Burnout. *Journal of Psychiatric Administration and Management*, 5(1), 13–15.

Monnat, S., & Chandler, R. (2014). Long term physical health consequences of adverse childhood experiences. Retrieved from http://paa2014.princeton.edu/papers/140160

Montesanti, S. R., & Thurston, W. E. (2015). Mapping the role of structural and interpersonal violence in the lives of women: Implications for public health interventions and policy. *BMC Women's Health*, 15(1), 100.

Murphy, M., Fiorillo, J., & Sullivan, A. (2014). The adverse childhood experiences (ACE) study and practice implications for attorneys for the child. Retrieved from https://ubir.buffalo.edu/xmlui/bitstream/handle/10477/25418/ACES%20Paper%20for%20AFC%20CLE.pdf

My Brother's Keeper. (2016). *My Brother's Keeper. 2016 progress report.* Retrieved from www.white house.gov/sites/whitehouse.gov/files/images/MBK-2016-Progress-Report.pdf

National Academy of Sciences. (2000). *From neurons to neighborhoods: The science of early childhood development.* Retrieved from www.ncbi.nlm.nih.gov/books/NBK225558/

National Academy of Sciences. (2014). *New directions in child abuse and neglect research.* Retrieved from www.ncbi.nlm.nih.gov/books/NBK195987/

National Child Traumatic Stress Network. (2017). *Addressing race and trauma in the classroom: A resource for educators.* Retrieved from https://youthlaw.org/wp-content/uploads/2017/09/FINAL-Race-a nd-Trauma-in-the-Classroom-Factsheet.pdf

National Scientific Council on the Developing Child. (2012). *Establishing a level foundation for life: Mental health begins in early childhood.* Retrieved from https://46y5eh11fhgw3ve3ytpwxt9r-wpengine.netdna -ssl.com/wp-content/uploads/2008/05/Establishing-a-Level-Foundation-for-Life-Mental-Hea lth-Begins-in-Early-Childhood.pdf

National Society for the Prevention of Cruelty to Children (NSPCC). (2016). *Child protection in England: Statistics.* Retrieved from www.nspcc.org.uk/preventing-abuse/child-protection-system/engla nd/statistics/

National Volunteer Caregiving Network (n.d.). Quotes from various cultures and faith traditions. Retrieved from https://nvcnetwork.org/wp/wp-content/uploads/2018/07/Quotes_from_Various_ Cultures_and_Faith_Traditions.pdf

Najavits, L. M. (2002). *Seeking safety: A treatment manual for PTSD and substance abuse.* New York: Guilford.

Niles, H., Mehta, D., Corrigan, A., Bhasin, M., & Denninger, J. (2014). Functional genomics in the study of mind-body therapies. *The Ochsner Journal*, 14(4), 681–695.

Nixon, L., Rodriguez, A., Han, S., Mejia, P., & Dorfman, L. (2017). Adverse childhood experiences in the news: Successes and opportunities in coverage of childhood trauma. *Public Health Institute.* Retrieved from www.phi.org/resources/?resource=adverse-childhood-experiences-in-the-news-successes-and-opportuni ties-in-coverage-of-childhood-trauma

Nixon, L., Somji, A., Mejia, P., Dorfman, L., & Quintero, F. (2015). Talking about trauma. Bmsg. Retrieved from www.bmsg.org/wp-content/uploads/2015/10/bmsg_talking_about_trauma_news_a nalysis2015.pdf

Noble, K. G. (2014). Rich man, poor man: Socioeconomic adversity and brain development. *Cerebrum: The Dana Forum on Brain Science*, 6, 1–12.

Noffsinger, M. A., Pfefferbaum, B., Pfefferbaum, R. L., Sherrieb, K., & Norris, F. H. (2012). The burden of disaster: Part I. Challenges and opportunities within a child's social ecology. *International Journal of Emergency Mental Health*, 14(1), 3–13.

Noonan, N. (2018). 6 more things we hope Oprah Winfrey covers about childhood trauma this Sunday night. *Institute for Attachment and Child Development.* Retrieved from https://www.institute forattachment.org/6-more-things-we-hope-oprah-winfrey-covers-about-childhood-trauma-this- sunday-night/

Nurius, P. S., Green, S., Logan-Greene, P., & Borja, S. (2015). Life course pathways of adverse childhood experiences toward adult psychological well-being: A stress process analysis. *Child Abuse & Neglect*, 45, 143–153.

Nurius, P. S., Prince, D. M., & Rocha, A. (2015). Cumulative disadvantage and youth well-being: A multi-domain examination with life course implications. *Child & Adolescent Social Work Journal*, 32(6), 567–576. doi:10.1007/s10560-015-0396-2

Office of Disease Prevention and Health Promotion. (2018). Social determinants of health. Retrieved from www.healthypeople.gov/2020/topics-objectives/topic/social-determinants-of-health

Ogle, C. M., Rubin, D. C., & Siegler, I. C. (2015). The relation between insecure attachment and posttraumatic stress: Early life versus adulthood traumas. *Psychological Trauma: Theory, Research, Practice and Policy*, 7(4), 324–332.

Olofson, M. (2017). Childhood adversity, families, neighborhoods, and cognitive outcomes: Testing structural models of the bioecological framework. *International Journal of Education and Practice*, 5(12), 199–216.

Oregon School-Based Health Alliance. (2017). *Dedicated to strengthening and sustaining Oregon's school-based health services.* Retrieved from http://osbha.org/files/OSBHA_general_brochure_FINAL.pdf

Osborne-Majnik, A., Fu, Q., & Lane, R. H. (2013). Epigenetic mechanisms in fetal origins of health and disease. *Clinical Obstetrics and Gynecology, 56*(3), 622–632.

Osher, D., Cantor, P., Berg, J., Steyer, L., & Rose, T. (2018). *Drivers of human development: How relationships and context shape learning and development.* Retrieved from https://assets.aspeninstitute.org/content/uploads/2017/12/Osher-Cantor-Berg-Steyer-Rose_Drivers-of-Human-Development_IN-PRESS.pdf

Osher, D., Cantor, P., Berg, J., Steyer, L., Rose, T., & Nolan, E. (2017). *Science of learning and development: A synthesis.* American Institutes for Research. Retrieved from https://assets.aspeninstitute.org/content/uploads/2017/09/pre-reading-Science-of-Learning-and-Development-Synthesis.pdf

Paccione-Dyszlewski, M. (2016). Trauma-informed schools: A must. *Brown University Child & Adolescent Behavior Letter, 32*(7), 8.

Padgett, D. K., Smith, B. T., Henwood, B. F., & Tiderington, E. (2012). Life course adversity in the lives of formerly homeless persons with serious mental illness: Context and meaning. *The American Journal of Orthopsychiatry, 82*(3), 421–430.

Pagani, M., Castelnuovo, G., Daverio, A., La Porta, P., Monaco, L., Ferrentino, F. … Di Lorenzo, G. (2018). Metabolic and electrophysiological changes associated to clinical improvement in two severely traumatized subjects treated with EMDR—A pilot study. *Frontiers in Psychology, 9,* 1–15. Retrieved from https://www.ncbi.nlm.nih.gov/pmc/articles/PMC5911467/

Paterson, S., Parish-Morris, J., Hirsh-Pasek, K., & Golinkoff, R. (2016). Considering development in developmental disorders. *Journal of Cognition and Development, 17*(4), 568–583.

Perreira, K., & Gallo, L. (2017). Adverse childhood experiences: Addressing health disparities through prevention, early detection and intervention. *American Heart Association.* Retrieved from https://professional.heart.org/professional/ScienceNews/UCM_498092_Adverse-Childhood-Experiences-Addressing-Health-Disparities-through-Prevention.jsp

Perry, D. F., & Conners-Burrow, N. (2016). Addressing early adversity through mental health consultation in early childhood settings. *Family Relations, 65*(1), 24–36.

Peters, J. & Silvestri, F. (2016). Healthy families: From ACEs to trauma informed care to resilience and wellbeing. Retrieved from http://www.iimhl.com/files/docs/Make_It_So/20161206.pdf

Phifer, L., & Hall, R. (2016). Helping students heal: Observations of trauma-informed practices in the schools. *School Mental Health, 8,* 201–205.

Philadelphia ACE Project (2019). History. Retrieved from http://philadelphiaaces.org/history

Philadelphia CeaseFire. (2014). A campaign to stop gun violence in our community: What is CeaseFire. Retrieved from www.philaceasefire.com/about.html

Philadelphia Higher Education Network for Neighborhood Development. (2014). Report from My Brother's Keeper task force. Retrieved from http://phennd.org/update/report-from-my-brothers-keeper-task-force/

Phillips, J. C., Parent, M. C., Dozier, C., & Jackson, P. L. (2016). Depth of discussion of multicultural identities in supervision and supervisory outcomes. *Counselling Psychology Quarterly, 30*(2), 188–210.

Pratchett, L. C., & Yehuda, R. (2011). Foundations of posttraumatic stress disorder: Does early life trauma lead to adult posttraumatic stress disorder? *Development and Psychopathology, 23,* 477–491.

Prevent child abuse (n.d.). Retrieved from www.preventchildabuse.org/images/docs/anda_wht_ppr.pdf

Purewal, S., Bucci, M., Wang, L., Koita, K., Marques, S., & Harris, N. (2016). Screening for adverse childhood experiences in an integrated pediatric model. *Zero to Three, 36*(3), 10–17.

Purtle, J., & Lewis, M. (2017). Mapping "trauma-informed" legislative proposals in U.S. congress. *Administration and Policy in Mental Health and Mental Health Services Research, 44*(6), 867–876.

Putnam, K. T., Harris, W. W., & Putnam, F. W. (2013). Synergistic childhood adversities and complex adult psychopathology. *Journal of Traumatic Stress, 26,* 435–442.

Pyle, J., Golderer, B., & Hargro, S. (2016). Trauma-informed philanthropy: Leveraging resources and relationships to advance trauma-informed practice and move from knowledge to action. Retrieved from https://philanthropynetwork.org/sites/default/files/Trauma2-web%20%281%29.pdf

Quiros, L., & Berger, R. (2015). Responding to the sociopolitical complexity of trauma: An integration of theory and practice. *Journal of Loss and Trauma*, 20(2), 149–159.

Racco, A., & Vis, J. (2015). Evidence based trauma treatment for children and youth. *Child & Adolescent Social Work Journal*, 32(2), 121–129.

Raising the Village. (2013). *Measuring the well-being of children and families in Toronto*. Retrieved from https://raisingthevillage.ca/wp-content/uploads/2017/12/Raising-the-Village-Part-2-Indigenous-Outcomes-April-2016-AODA.pdf

Raja, S., Hasnain, M., Hoersch, M., Gove-Yin, S., & Rajagopalan, C. (2015). Trauma informed care in medicine. Current knowledge and future research directions. *Family & Community Health*, 38(3), 216–226. Retrieved from http://floridatrauma.org/Resources/TIC_InMedicine.pdf

Ramos-Olazagasti, M., Bird, H., Canino, G. J., & Duarte, C. S. (2017). Childhood adversity and early initiation of alcohol use in two representative samples of Puerto Rican youth. *Journal of Youth and Adolescence*, 46(1), 28–44.

Rantin, B. (2014, August 22). Celebrating a legacy of protecting children. *The State*. Retrieved from www.thestate.com/news/local/article13877663.html.

Rhodes, J. (2015). The chronicle of evidence based mentoring. The William Grant Foundation. Retrieved from www.evidencebasedmentoring.org/the-william-t-grant-foundation-releases-a-new-report-on-disparities-in-youths-use-of-health-and-mental-health-services-in-the-u-s/

Rich, J., Corbin, T., Bloom, S., Rich, L., Evans, S., & Wilson, A. (2009). Healing the hurt: Trauma-informed approaches to the health of boys and young men of color. Drexel University College of Medicine. Retrieved from www.unnaturalcauses.org/assets/uploads/file/HealingtheHurt-Trauma-Rich%20et%20al.pdf

Rogers, B. (2015). *Trauma & resilience. Informed Solutions Institute of Southern Africa. Proposal of a trauma-activist*. PTG-RR. Retrieved from www.ptgrr.com/images/TRISI%20Section%2011.%20Resilience%20and%20Trauma%204.pdf

Romens, S. E., McDonald, J., Svaren, J., & Pollak, S. D. (2015). Associations between early life stress and gene methylation in children. *Child Development*, 86, 303–309.

Sabo, S., Shaw, S., Ingram, M., Teufel-Shone, N., Carvajal, S., de Zapien, J., & Rubio-Goldsmith, R. (2014). Everyday violence, structural racism and mistreatment at the US-Mexico border. *Social Science & Medicine*, 109, 66–74.

Sacks, V., & Murphey, D. (2018). The prevalence of adverse childhood experiences, nationally, by state, and by race or ethnicity. *Child Trends*. Retrieved from www.childtrends.org/publications/prevalence-adverse-childhood- experiences-nationally-state-race-ethnicity

Safe & Sound. (2018). The economics of child abuse. Retrieved from https://safeandsound.org/economics-child-abuse-study-san-francisco/

Salloum, A., Johnco, C., Smyth, K., Murphy, T. & Storch, A. (2018). Co-Occurring posttraumatic stress disorder and depression among young children. *Child Psychiatry & Human Development*, 49(3), 452–459.

SAMHSA: Project Aware. (2017). Measuring progress towards becoming a trauma-informed school. Retrieved from www.nhstudentwellness.org/uploads/5/3/9/0/53900547/measuring_trauma_informed_schools_11.10.17.pdf

San Francisco's Trauma Informed Systems Initiative. (2014). *Trauma informed system initiative*. San Francisco Department of Public Health. Retrieved from www.leapsf.org/pdf/Trauma-Informed-Systems-Initative-2014.pdf

Sansbury, B. S., Graves, K., & Scott, W. (2015). Managing traumatic stress responses among clinicians: Individual and organizational tools for self-care. *Trauma*, 17(2), 114–122.

School-Based Health Alliance. (2017). National school-based healthcare census. Retrieved from www.sbh4all.org/school-health-care/national-census-of-school-based-health-centers/

Shaffer, C., Smith, T., & Ornstein, A. (2018). Child and youth advocacy centres: A change in practice that can change a lifetime. *Paediatrics & Child Health*, 23(2), 116–118.

Shonkoff, J., Garner, A., The Committee on Pychosocial Aspects of Child and Family Health, Committee on Early Childhood Adoption and Dependent Care, and Section on Developmental and

Behavioral Pediatrics, Siegel, B. ...Wood, L. (2012). The lifelong effects of early childhood adversity and toxic stress. *Pediatrics*, 129(1), e232–e246.

Skousen, T. (n.d.). *Native American resilience*. Retrieved from http://resilitator.com/pdf/NativeAmerica nResilience_TSkousen.pdf

Slopen, N., Shonkoff, J., Albert, M., Yoshikawa, H., Jacobs, A., Stoltz, R., & Williams, D. (2016). Racial disparities in child adversity in the U.S.: Interactions with family immigration history and income. *American Journal of Preventive Medicine*, 50(1), 47–56.

Smith, A. (2016). Achieving social justice for children: How can children's rights thinking make a difference? *American Journal of Orthopsychiatry*, 86(5), 500–507.

Smith, C. A., Park, A., Ireland, T. O., Elwyn, L., & Thornberry, T. (2013). Long-term outcomes of young adults exposed to maltreatment: The role of educational experiences in promoting resilience to crime and violence in early adulthood. *Journal of Interpersonal Violence*, 28(1), 121–156.

Snyder, R., & Lyon, N. (2017). *Becoming trauma informed: A guide for child serving programs and organizations*. Michigan Department of Health & Human Services. Retrieved from www.michigan.gov/documents/mdhhs/Becoming_Trauma_Informed_576292_7.pdf

Soleimanpour, S., Geierstanger, S., & Brindis, C. (2017). Adverse childhood experiences and resilience: Addressing the unique needs of adolescents. *Academic Pediatrics*, 17, S108–S114.

Steinberg, J., & Lassiter, W. (2018). Toward a trauma-responsive juvenile justice system. *North Carolina Medical Journal*, 79(2), 115–118.

Stiles, S. (2003). Severe obesity. *The Permanente Journal*, 7(2), 49–52. Retrieved from www.thepermanentejournal.org/files/Spring2003/severe.pdf

Strait, J., & Bolman, T. (2017). Consideration of personal adverse childhood experiences during implementation of trauma-informed care curriculum in graduate health programs. *The Permanente Journal*, 21, 16–61.

Stouthamer-Loeber, M., Loeber, R., Homish, D., & Wei, E. (2001). Maltreatment of boys and the development of disruptive and delinquent behavior. *Developmental Psychopathology*, 13(4), 941–955.

Stroud, L. R., Papandonatos, G. D., Rodriguez, D., McCallum, M., Salisbury, A. L., Phipps, M. G. ... Marsit, C. J. (2014). Maternal smoking during pregnancy and infant stress response: Test of a prenatal programming hypothesis. *Psychoneuroendocrinology*, 48, 29–40.

Substance Abuse and Mental Health Services Administration (SAMHSA). (2014). *Trauma- informed care in behavioral health services: A treatment improvement protocol* (TIP 57), HHS Publication No. (SMA) 14–4816. Rockville, MD: U.S. Department of Health and Human Services. SAMHSA.

Sykes, B., Piquero, A., & Gioviano, J. (2017). Code of the classroom? Social disadvantage and bullying among A00merican adolescents, U.S. 2011–2012. *Crime & Delinquency*, 63(14) 1883–1922.

Szyf, M., & Meaney, M. (2008). Epigenetics, behaviour, and health. *Allergy, Asthma, and Clinical Immunology*, 4(1), 37–49.

Szyf, M., Tang, Y.-Y., Hill, K. G., & Musci, R. (2016). The dynamic epigenome and its implications for behavioral interventions: A role for epigenetics to inform disorder prevention and health promotion. *Translational Behavioral Medicine*, 6(1), 55–62.

Tam, T. W., Zlotnick, C., & Robertson, M. J. (2003). Longitudinal perspective: Adverse childhood events, substance use, and labor force participation among homeless adults. *American Journal of Drug and Alcohol Abuse*, 29(4), 829–846.

Texas Care for Children. (2017). Student mental health after the storm. Retrieved from https://static1.squarespace.com/static/5728d34462cd94b84dc567ed/t/5a26c2bfe2c483d3d36df817/1512489667626/after-the-storm.pdf

The Commonwealth (2017). *Preventing violence, promoting peace*. Retrieved from https://srhr- ask-us.org/wp-content/uploads/2018/04/Preventing-Violence-Main-PolicyToolkit.pdf

Therapist Certification Program. (2018). Trauma-Focused Cognitive Behavioral Therapy-(TF-CBT). Retrieved from www.tfcbt.org

Thompson-Lastad, A., Yen, I., Fleming, M., Natta, M., Rubin, S., & Burke, N. (2017). Defining trauma in complex care management: Safety-net providers' perspectives on structural vulnerability and time. *Social Science & Medicine*, 186, 104–112.

Tomer, J. (2014). Adverse childhood experiences, poverty, and inequality: Toward an understanding of the connections and the cures. *World Economic Review*, 3, 20–36.

Trauma Informed Philanthropy. (2016). A funder's resource guide for supporting trauma-informed practice in the Delaware Valley. Retrieved from https://c.ymcdn.com/sites/www.philanthropynet work.org/resource/resmgr/pn_miscdocs/TraumaGUIDE_FinalWeb.pdf

Travis, R. (2017). All awareness and no action: Can social work leverage creative arts' potential? *Research on Social Work Practice*, 1–3. Retrieved from www.researchgate.net/profile/Raphael_Travis/publication/320912839_All_Aware ness_and_No_Action_Can_Social_Work_Leverage_Creative_Arts%27_Potential/links/5ab52f29aca2722b97ca2888/All-Awareness-and-No-Action-Can-Social-Work-Leverage-Creative-Arts-Potential.pdf

Turner, S. (2009). *Exploring resilience in the lives of women leaders in early childhood health, human services, and education*. PhD thesis. Oregon State University. (Order No. 3385620). Available from ProQuest Dissertations & Theses Global. (304976716).

Tyrka, A. R., Ridout, K. K., Parade, S. H., Paquette, A., Marsit, C. J., & Seifer, R. (2015). Childhood maltreatment and methylation of FKBP5. *Development and Psychopathology*, 27(4 Pt 2), 1637–1645. http://doi.org/10.1017/S0954579415000991

UK Parliament. (2018). The evidence behind early intervention. Retrieved from https://publications.pa rliament.uk/pa/cm201719/cmselect/cmsctech/506/50605.htm

Umberson, D. (2017). Black deaths matter: Race, relationship loss, and effects on survivors. *Journal of Health and Social Behavior*, 58(4) 405–420.

Ungar, M. (2015). Practitioner review: Diagnosing childhood resilience –a systemic approach to the diagnosis of adaptation in adverse social and physical ecologies. *Journal of Child Psychology and Psychiatry*, 56(1), 4–17.

United Nations Development Programme (UNDP). (2014). *Human development report 2014. Sustaining human progress: Reducing vulnerabilities and building resilience*. Retrieved from http://hdr.undp.org/sites/default/files/hdr14-report-en-1.pdf

University of Buffalo. (2018). Trauma informed certificate programs. Retrieved from http://socialwork.buffalo.edu/continuing-education/certificate-programs/trauma.html

US Department of Health and Human Services (US DHHS) (2015). *Administration for children and families, administration on children, youth and families. Child maltreatment 2013*. Retrieved from www.acf.hhs.gov/programs/cb/resource/child- maltreatment- 2013.

Usman, C. (2016). *Addressing homelessness and health inequalities through community development*. University of Northern British Columbia. Retrieved from https://core.ac.uk/download/pdf/84871613.pdf

Vaisvaser, S., Modai, S., Farberov, L., Lin, T., Sharon, H., Gilam, A., ... Hendler, T. (2016). Neuro-epigenetic indications of acute stress response in humans: The case of MicroRNA- 29c. *PLoS One*, 11(1), e0146236.

Valentino, K. (2017). Relational interventions for maltreated children. *Child Development*, 88(2), 359–367.

van Dijken, M.W., Stams, G.J.J.M., & de Winter, M., (2016). Can community-based interventions prevent child maltreatment?, Children and Youth Services Review, 61(C), 149–158.

van IJzendoorn, M. H., Bakermans-Kranenburg, M. J., & Ebstein, R. P. (2011). Methylation matters in child development: Toward developmental behavioral epigenetics. *Child Development Perspectives*, 5(4), 305–310.

Varghese, R., Quiros, L., & Berger, R. (2018). Reflective practices for engaging in trauma- informed culturally competent supervision. *Smith College Studies in Social Work*. 88(2), 135–151. Retrieved from https://doi.org/10.1080/00377317.2018.1439826

Vermont Department of Health. (2014). *Childhood trauma and its impact on community wellness*. Retrieved from www.healthvermont.gov/sites/default/files/documents/2016/11/OLH_Childhood_Trauma_a nd_Its_Impact_On_Community_Wellness.pdf

Wade, R., Cronholm, P. F., Fein, J. A., Forke, C. M., Davis, M. B., Harkins-Schwarz, M. ... Bair-Merritt, M. H. (2016). Household and community-level adverse childhood experiences and adult health outcomes in a diverse urban population. *Child Abuse and Neglect*, 52, 135–145.

Wade, R., Shea, J., Rubin, D., & Wood, J. (2014). Adverse childhood experiences of low-income urban youth. *Pediatrics*, 134(1), e13–e20.

Wagner, J. R., Busche, S., Ge, B., Kwan, T., Pastinen, T., & Blanchette, M. (2014). The relationship between DNA methylation, genetic and expression inter-individual variation in untransformed human fibroblasts. *Genome Biology*, 15(2), R37. Retrieved from http://doi.org/10.1186/gb-2014-15-2-r37

Walsh, M., & Theodorakakis, M. (2017). The impact of economic inequality on children's development and achievement. *Religions*, 8(4), 67.

Watkins, C. E. (2014). Clinical supervision in the 21st century: Revisiting pressing needs and impressing possibilities. *American Journal of Psychotherapy*, 68(2), 251–272.

Weinreb, L., Savageau, J. A., Candib, L. M., Reed, G. W., Fletcher, K. E., & Hargraves, J. L. (2010). Screening for childhood trauma in adult primary care patients: A cross-sectional survey. *Primary Care Companion to the Journal of Clinical Psychiatry*, 12(6), 1–18. doi:10.4088/PCC.10m00950blu

Wessells, M. (2015). A social environment approach to promotive and protective practice in childhood resilience: Reflections on Ungar. *Journal of Child Psychology & Psychiatry*, 56(1),18–20.

West, J. (2014). *The role of social work in contemporary colonial and structurally violent processes: Speaking to aboriginal social workers who had child welfare and/or criminal justice involvement as youth.* PhD thesis. University of Manitoba. Retrieved from https://mspace.lib.umanitoba.ca/bitstream/handle/1993/23854/West%20Juliana.pdf?sequence=3

Wheeler, K. (2018). A call for trauma competencies in nursing education. *Journal of the American Psychiatric Nurses Association*, 24(1), 20–22. Retrieved from http://journals.sagepub.com/doi/full/10.1177/1078390317745080

Widener University. (2018). On line Masters of Social Work program. Retrieved from https://onlineprograms.widener.edu/msw/masters-of-social-work

Widom, C. S., DuMont, K., & Czaja, S. J. (2007). A prospective investigation of major depressive disorder and comorbidity in abused and neglected children grown up. *Archives of General Psychiatry*, 64(1), 49–56.

Williams, S. (2016). *The role of problem behaviors in the pathway from abuse to prostitution.* PhD thesis. Walden University. Retrieved from https://scholarworks.waldenu.edu/cgi/viewcontent.cgi?article=3241&context=dissertations

Wilson, F. (2016). Identifying, preventing, and addressing job burnout and vicarious burnout for social work professionals. *Journal of Evidence-Informed Social Work*, 13(5), 479–483.

Winfrey, O. (2018, March 11). Treating childhood trauma. *CBS News: 60 minutes.* Retrieved from www.cbsnews.com/news/oprah-winfrey-treating-childhood-trauma/

Wu, Y., Dissing-Olesen, L., MacVicar, B. A., & Stevens, B. (2015). Microglia: Dynamic mediators of synapse development and plasticity. *Trends in Immunology*, 36(10), 605–613.

Yang, X., Han, H., De Carvalho, D. D., Lay, F. D., Jones, P. A., & Liang, G. (2014). Gene body methylation can alter gene expression and is a therapeutic target in cancer. *Cancer Cell*, 26(4), 577–590.

Yaroshefsky, E., & Shwedel, A. (2015). Changing the school to prison pipeline: Integrating trauma informed care in the New York City school system, in *Collected essays. Impact: Threat of Economic Inequality*, 1, 99. Retrieved from https://scholarlycommons.law.hofstra.edu/faculty_scholarship/918

Zmijewski, C. (2014). *Positive neuroplasticity improves brain and body health.* Retrieved from www.ptonthenet.com/articles/positive-neuroplasticity-improves-brain-and-body-health-3917

INDEX

Page locators in *italics* indicate figures and boxes; locators in **bold** indicate tables

Printed in the United States
by Baker & Taylor Publisher Services